C000133676

Shared Care

Asthma

Shared Care for Asthma

Mark L. Levy MBChB FRCGP
General Practitioner, Harrow, Middlesex;
Editor of *Asthma in General Practice* and Medical Advisor,
National Asthma and Respiratory Training Centre, Warwick, UK

Jon M. Couriel MA FRCP FRCPCH
Consultant in Paediatric Respiratory Medicine,
Booth Hall Children's Hospital,
University of Manchester, UK

Roland A. Clark BSc MBChB FRCP
Consultant Physician and Senior Lecturer,
University of Dundee,
Dundee Teaching Hospitals NHS Trust,
Dundee, UK

Stephen T. Holgate BSc MBBS MD DSc FRCP FRCP(E)
Clinical Professor of Immunopharmacology,
University Medicine, Southampton General Hospital, UK

Anoop J. Chauhan MBChB MRCP
MRC Training Fellow,
Faculty of Medicine, University of Southampton,
Southampton General Hospital, UK

I S I S
MEDICAL
M E D I A
—
Oxford

© 1997 Isis Medical Media Ltd
58 St Aldates
Oxford OX1 1ST, UK

First published 1997

British Library Cataloguing in Publication Data
A catalogue record for this title is available from the British Library

ISBN 1 899066 41 1

Levy, M (Mark)
Shared Care for Asthma
Mark Levy, Jon Couriel, Roland Clark, Stephen Holgate and Anoop Chauhan

Always refer to the manufacturer's Prescribing Information before prescribing drugs cited in this book.

Illustrated by
Suzanne Benjamin

Typeset by
Creative Associates, Oxford, UK

Printed and bound by
Jarrold Book Printing, Thetford, UK

Distributed in the USA by
Mosby-Year Book Inc.,
11830 Westline Industrial Drive,
St Louis, Mo 63145, USA

Distributed in the rest of the world by
Oxford University Press, Saxon Way West,
Corby, Northamptonshire NN18 9ES, UK

Contents

Foreword

Asthma is one of the commonest chronic diseases and, even by conservative estimates, there are approximately three million sufferers in the United Kingdom. The majority of these have relatively mild asthma and are eminently suitable for management in the community. However, most surveys suggest that around 15% of those with asthma also require hospital care at some time. This represents a significant proportion of hospital and A&E department workload, and admissions for acute asthma are among the most frequent medical emergencies. In recent years, changes in health care and health policy have led to an increasing shift of emphasis from the hospital base to a community base. The 'primary–secondary care interface' is a jargon term which has now become accepted by all those working in health care, and it identifies the area where much innovative service development is occurring. This requires collaborative approaches between primary care health professionals and hospital specialists, and this book, therefore, is a timely contribution to our understanding of present good practice in shared care for asthma.

In particular, Chapter 3 summarizes effectively the massive advances made over the past ten years in our understanding of the basic mechanisms of asthma. There are helpful reviews of the areas of diagnosis and management. The structural changes in general practice over the past ten years have led to great improvements in the organization of care for those with asthma, and this book gives a state of the art review of this, including the pivotal role of the nurse run asthma clinic in general practice. Those patients discharged from hospital after acute asthma are a particularly important group which requires the best possible collaborative arrangements for follow-up. The final chapter contains a series of challenging case studies which illustrate the important issues in planning effective shared care.

Mark Levy and his co-authors are to be congratulated on this important and comprehensive textbook.

Sean Hilton MD FRCGP
Professor of General Practice and Primary Care,
St. George's Hospital Medical School, University of London

Preface

Shared Care for Asthma was written to explore the interface between the different sectors (community and hospital) responsible for asthma care and to raise questions and issues which may serve to promote shared care between these sectors. This book is intended for busy health care professionals involved in the care of asthma patients, but it is not intended to be a complete text on the subject.

Why this book? Problems arise when patients move within the sectors of health care because of the difficulties in maintaining continuity of care. For example, asthma patients attending their family practitioner may see a different doctor each time they attend during a specific period of illness. Similarly, in the hospital sector, with the 4–6 monthly rotation of junior staff, patients attending over a long period of time may be cared for by many different doctors.

The authors of this book share an abiding interest in asthma care, but mostly in their own spheres of influence. Jon Couriel is a specialist respiratory paediatrician, Roland Clark a respiratory adult physician, Stephen Holgate and Anoop Chauhan are involved at the forefront of clinical pharmacology research, particularly in the respiratory field, and Mark Levy is a family practitioner with a special interest in asthma. The dialogue about shared care that has ensued, and which follows on the pages of this book, has not been an easy undertaking, perhaps reflecting the difficulties experienced by us all in managing this common, but complex respiratory disease.

The contents of the book range from a description of the pathogenesis and molecular mechanisms of the disease, through practical aspects of care and management of asthma in the community and the hospital, to individual illustrative case histories. We start with an introductory chapter which is followed by a description of the extent of the problems in terms of prevalence, morbidity, mortality and issues related to organization and economics of asthma care. Chapter 3 addresses the mechanisms of asthma development and relates these, where possible, to the therapeutic approaches currently adopted by clinicians. Chapter 4 is about diagnosis of asthma with some ideas for improving the accuracy and speed with which the condition is recognized and confirmed. Then we discuss management of acute and chronic care of asthma, in adults and children, across the interface of primary through tertiary care, with examples of treatment charts from the latest update from the British Guidelines on asthma care. Chapter 6 describes the current organization of asthma care across the interface in the UK and offers suggestions for improvements in this area. The final chapter offers examples of case histories to illustrate some of the problems experienced by patients and health care professionals involved in asthma care across the interface.

M.L. Levy, J.M. Couriel, R.A. Clark, S.T. Holgate, A.J. Chauhan

Chapter 1

The concept

What is shared care?

Shared care in asthma is the joint management of patients and their families by primary, secondary and tertiary health care professionals. These include trained practice, community and hospital nurses; family practitioners, general paediatricians and adult physicians, as well as specialist adult and paediatric respiratory physicians and nurses. The diagnosis and management of asthma occurs across this spectrum of expertise and patients may require the services of some or many of these health professionals as the severity of their disease fluctuates during their lives.

The scope of the problem

Asthma affects the lives of about 7% of the population in the UK directly, and a considerable number of family members indirectly. Workload in the community and hospitals has increased substantially over the last two decades

The challenge

The challenge is to evolve a strategy that leads to early initial diagnosis, subsequent recognition of uncontrolled asthma and appropriate management of the patient. Communication across the interface may enhance this, for example if Accident and Emergency (A&E) departments notify GPs of recurrent attenders. By teaching patients and providing them with written self-management plans, early recognition of uncontrolled asthma may be improved. This should result in early intervention both in the form of initial therapy and in preventing acute attacks. In addition, scarce health resources need to be used efficiently by patients and health professionals. In order to achieve this goal, general awareness of the presenting features of asthma needs to be raised, perhaps by approaches such as that of the National Asthma Campaign's surgery poster which alerts people to the three major presenting symptoms of asthma (cough, wheeze and shortness of breath). The aim of this effort was to encourage patients and parents to present themselves to the doctor or nurse with the question: 'Have I got asthma?' Health professionals, on the other hand, need to raise their index of suspicion of asthma when consulted by patients with respiratory symptoms.

Asthmatic patients may attend different sectors of the health service at different times. Under these circumstances, care may become fragmented with lack of continuity as well as consistency. Therefore, ideally, a cohesive, continuous and seamless transition between the different sectors of the health service is desirable in order to provide the best care.

Most of the time, provided the patients' asthma is reasonably well controlled, routine follow-up consultations take place in primary care where the patients consult the GP or practice nurse with relatively easy access. Likewise, they usually attend the primary care health professionals in the first instance when their asthma goes out of control. However, there are times when referral (either by self or by the doctor or nurse) to secondary care is necessary. Under these circumstances, we suggest ideas for a formalized pre-agreed plan of action by the referring and receiving health professionals.

Continuity of care in asthmatic patients is important and this book aims to promote this by organized care and follow-up protocols. While this book is not meant to be a comprehensive text on the subject of asthma, great care has been taken to include the latest evidence-based information. All chapters are fully referenced so that the reader may delve deeper into areas of asthma theory if desired.

We believe that by adopting a shared care approach to the management of asthma, everyone will benefit, i.e. our patients and health professionals in primary care, the school medical service and hospital practice.

Chapter 2

Asthma: an overview

Asthma is one of the commonest chronic conditions. It affects people of all ages and places a significant economic burden on health-care resources. It is caused by a variety of triggers and varies in intensity over time. Patients consult health professionals with symptoms ranging from mild and infrequent to persistent disabling breathlessness. The mean prevalence of asthma in the UK is between 4 and 6%[1]. The distribution of prevalence by age varies considerably: approximately 15% of UK school children have asthma[2].

The morbidity associated with poorly controlled asthma is not only a burden for the individual patient but has a major impact on family, domestic and social life. Asthmatic children may:

■ face problems at school due to regularly disturbed sleep[3]
■ have difficulty in taking part in group activities
■ have their career opportunities limited and
■ suffer from emotional problems[4,5].

Parents of asthmatic children have their social life disrupted and, in a recent survey, 69% had lost time off work due to their child's asthma[6].

The financial burden of asthma upon the NHS, for the provision of care, sickness and invalidity benefits, is estimated to lie between 400 and 500 million pounds per annum[7,8]. In 1990 the prescription of bronchodilator and prophylactic medication accounted for 9% of the Scottish Drug Budget[9]. Between 1 September 1991 and 31 August 1992 more patients consulted their general practitioner for respiratory

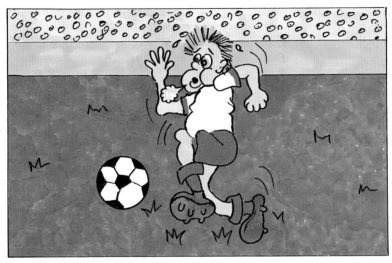

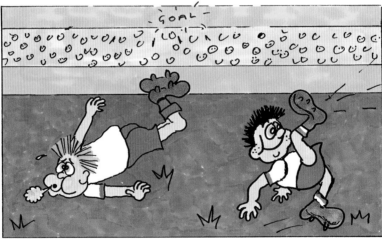

problems than for any other condition listed in the International Classification of Diseases (ICD): 30% people consulted at least once for a disease of the respiratory system; about 5% of all patients consulted for chronic obstructive pulmonary disease (COPD) — 80% of these were for asthma[10].

In this chapter the nature and presentation of asthma is discussed together with a review of problems relating to morbidity and mortality, the delivery of care and the relevant health economic factors.

What is asthma?

Due to the complex nature of asthma, clinicians have struggled to define the condition for over one hundred years[11-14]. It has been difficult to agree on a definition of asthma that is acceptable to all health workers and that takes into account the varying nature of patients' symptoms, the diverse natural history, the heterogeneity of the trigger factors as well as embracing the pathological features. The advent of fibreoptic bronchoscopy has allowed the pathogenesis of asthma to be investigated. It is now clear that, even in mild asthma, the inflammatory process is present. It is, however, necessary to have a working definition of asthma and we have

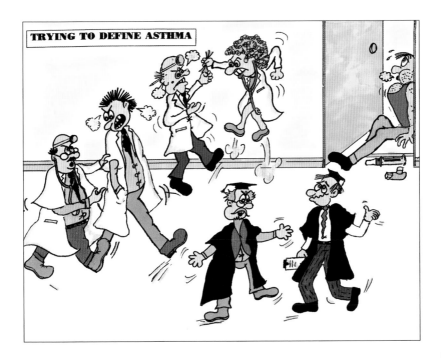

chosen to use the one used by the Global Initiative for Asthma (GINA):

"Asthma is a chronic inflammatory disorder of the airways. In susceptible individuals this inflammation causes recurrent episodes of coughing, wheezing, chest tightness and difficult breathing. Inflammation makes the airways sensitive to stimuli such as allergens, chemical irritants, tobacco smoke, cold air or exercise. When exposed to these stimuli, the airways may become swollen, constricted, filled with mucus and hyperresponsive to a variety of stimuli. The resulting airflow limitation is reversible (but not completely so in some patients), either spontaneously or with treatment. When asthma therapy is adequate, inflammation can be reduced over the long term, symptoms can be controlled and most asthma-related problems prevented[15]."

What causes asthma?

There is a complex interrelationship between genetic factors, atopy, bronchial reactivity, environmental factors and asthma. There is no clear indication as to why some individuals develop asthma while others with a similar constitutional make-up and exposed to the same external conditions do not. Atopy is not synonymous with asthma, but there is a close association between eczema, rhinitis and asthma[16].

Environmental factors implicated in the induction of asthma

- Allergens
- Smoking
- Infection
- Pollution
- Occupation
- Weather (temperature/humidity)

Allergens

While 40% of normal individuals have a positive skin test to common allergens without developing an atopic disorder[17], there is evidence that exposure increases the risk of children generating a sensitivity to dust mite allergen followed by asthma[18]. The level of exposure to house dust mite antigen during the first year of life has been shown to be a major factor determining whether a child born to atopic parents will develop asthma, there being a close correlation between the level of antigen exposure[18] and the age of onset[19]. However, measures to reduce exposure to mite antigen and avoidance of dietary allergens in babies born to atopic mothers have been shown to reduce significantly the prevalence of eczema and allergy but not asthma[20].

Smoking

Maternal smoking in pregnancy have been shown to be associated with an increased risk of atopy, raised cord blood IgE levels and reduced lung function in children when compared with babies born to non-smoking mothers. Passive (involuntary) smoking in early childhood, particularly maternal smoking, is associated with an increased risk of developing asthma, with earlier onset and greater severity of symptoms[21,22]. Since World War II, maternal smoking has increased dramatically and is considered a possible factor in the increased prevalence and severity of childhood asthma.

Infections

Viral infections cause transient increased bronchial hyperreactivity in atopic and non-atopic individuals. However, there is insufficient evidence at present to confirm that viruses initiate the development of asthma[23], although viral infections are a common trigger factor.

Pollutants and the environment

Atmospheric pollutants such as ozone, sulphur dioxide and the oxides of nitrogen by themselves are unlikely to cause asthma, although they may act in conjunction with allergens in sensitizing the human airway. However, once asthma is established there is no doubt that these agents can exacerbate symptoms and patients should heed media warnings of poor air quality and take appropriate action. Recently interest has focused on the role of pollutants in local epidemics of asthma such as those which occurred in Barcelona as a result of atmospheric pollution from soya bean dust[24] and in Britain[25,26] and Australia[27] in relation to electric thunder storms. These reports support the hypothesis that epidemics may be related to increased aeroallergens[28].

Occupation

Currently there are over 200 known respiratory sensitizers used in industry. Occupational asthma is discussed further in Chapter 5.

How common is asthma?

The differences in the definition of asthma and the methodology used between studies make it difficult to establish clearly the prevalence of asthma in Britain and how it may have changed over the last 20 years. Epidemiological studies rely largely on patients' self-reported asthma symptoms and their results vary according to the nature of the population surveyed, the questions asked and the response rate.

In Table 2.1 the disparity between results obtained using different methods, time scales, ages and assessment criteria, is well shown in a selection of studies. Using case notes, Gellert[29] showed a cumulative incidence of both diagnosed and wheezy episodes of 19.5% but an annual prevalence of only 9.3% whereas Jones[30] showed a cumulative prevalence of diagnosed asthma of 8.8%, using a questionnaire.

Several studies showing differences between populations and geographical areas have come from the Third World involving people of the same genetic stock. Studies comparing Xhosa children in Cape Town and the Transkei[36], the rural and urban populations in the Gambia[37] and highland and coastal regions in New Guinea[38] have all shown a higher prevalence of asthma amongst those living in higher economically developed areas. A Scottish study in 12-year-old children failed to show differences in urban and rural prevalence of asthma or wheeze, though there were differences in exercise-induced symptoms[39].

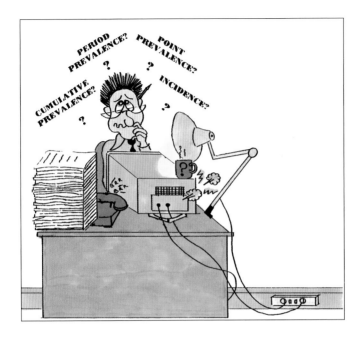

In the Tayside Childhood Asthma Study, a nurse facilitator, trained to review the general practice medical records of all children aged 1–15 from 10 representative practices, identified asthma-related features recorded during the child's lifetime. In the 10 460 notes reviewed, the cumulative prevalence of asthma was 8.4%, wheezy bronchitis 4.6% and recurrent bronchospasm 11.3%. Twenty percent had been prescribed anti-asthma treatment at some stage during their lives. The annual prevalence of asthma in this population was 10%[40].

Recent data from a study investigating the effect of training nurses to care for people with asthma provided information on the prevalence of diagnosed asthma in 466 general practices serving a population of more than 3 million people[41]. There were 209 612 patients (6.9%) diagnosed as asthmatic and Table 2.2 shows the distribution of mean prevalence of diagnosed asthma by sex and age. These figures are higher than those quoted nationally[42] and may reflect the relatively high level of asthma interest in these practices.

Table 2.1 Prevalence of asthma wheeze and related symptoms in children; some selected studies

Date	Method	Type of prevalence	Criteria	Age	Prevalence (%)
1983[30,31]	Q	Ann.	Wheeze	5	11.0
1984[32]	Audit	Cum.	Rx response/ PEF	2–11	11
1986[33]	Audit	Cum.	Rx response/ PEF	0–16	16
1990[29]	C/N	Ann.	Diagnosis/ wheeze	0–15	9.3
1990[29]	C/N	Cum.	Diagnosis/ wheeze	0–15	19.5
1990[34]	Q	Cum.	Diagnosis	0–12	8.8
1992[35]	I	Cum.	Diagnosis	11	21.8

Ann. = Annual; Cum. = Cumulative; C/N = Case notes; I = Interview; Q = Questionnaire.

Table 2.2 Distribution of mean prevalence of diagnosed asthma by sex and age in a population of over 3 million people served by 466 general practices[41] (n = 209612, percentages are shown)

Sex	Age (years)					
	<5	5–14	15–44	45–54	55–64	>65
Male	6.8	12.4	5.6	3.8	4.9	5.9
Female	4.4	9.3	5.9	5.1	5.9	5.2

Evidence showing a rise in prevalence of asthma has been more difficult to obtain. However, there does appear to be a real upward trend over the last 30 years[23]. Two studies in Aberdeen school children, 25 years apart, involving the same population and using similar methods, were recently compared. They showed a doubling of self-reported wheeze from 10.9 to 19.8% and a rise in the diagnosis of asthma from 4.1 to 10.2%. The prevalence of wheezing not diagnosed as asthma increased from 7.5 to 9.8%. This suggests that the true prevalence of asthma has increased[43].

In the late 1970s it was estimated that 4.5% of the population were regularly consulting their general practitioners for asthma symptoms; today these consultation rates are in the region of 6–7%. The weekly return service for the Royal College of General Practitioners shows a rise in consultations for asthma from 8–12 per 100 000 population in 1976 to 40–50 in 1994[44]. The increase in consultation rates affects all ages[44] but is more marked in the younger age groups as seen in Figure 2.1[42].

Figure 2.1 illustrates the growing workload for asthma (from 1984 to 1993) carried by general practitioners, whether this is due to increased prevalence, increased awareness or better diagnosis, particularly as the assessment and medication of asthmatic patients is more time-consuming than for many other ailments.

In a postal survey of 6000 people aged 20–40 in Scotland 650 reported wheeze continuing over 2 years. 42% had not contacted their GP in the last year including 68% who reported symptoms severe enough to interfere with normal daily activities[1]. These data suggest that there may be as many as 23 000 people (1.2% of the Scottish population aged 20–44) suffering from significant morbidity from asthma-like symptoms who are not attending their GPs. Underdiagnosis remains an important factor in asthma management.

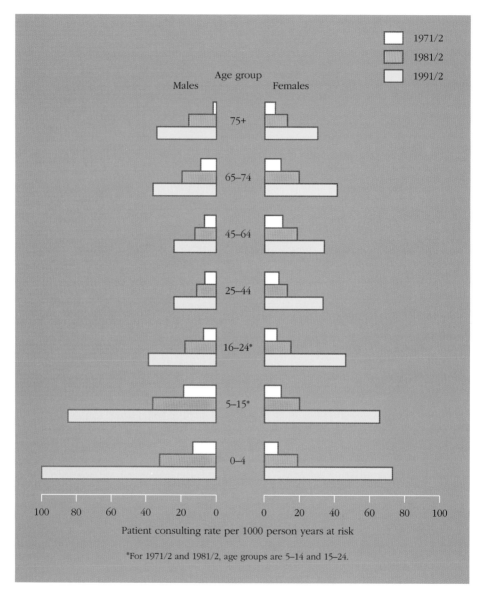

Figure 2.1 *Patients consulting their GP for asthma by sex and age, England and Wales
1971/72, 1981/82, 1991/92.
Source: Morbidity Statistics from General Practice 1991/92, 1995.
Crown Copyright 1995. Reproduced by permission of the Controller of HMSO and the
Office for National Statistics.*

Natural history of asthma

Pattern of disease

Wheezing illness seen by health professionals is commoner at the extremes of life (Figure 2:1); 80% of children with asthma develop symptoms before the age of 5. Asthma is twice as common and symptoms start earlier in prepubertal boys but the sex differential is lost during adolescence. By middle age the incidence is higher in females.

Do children 'grow out' of their asthma? The National Childhood Development Study showed a rapid decline in the prevalence of reported wheeze from 8.3% at the age 7 to 4.7% by the age of 11 and 3.5% at 16. Only 10.5% reporting wheeze had persistent symptoms in each age group. The more severe the symptoms at the age of 7, the more likely they are to persist into teenage years[45]. However, when followed-up for a longer period, patients who appeared to have grown out of their asthma reported that they had relapsed and developed symptoms[16]. The most comprehensive longitudinal case study (from Australia) of childhood asthma showed that:

- by the age of 21, only 32% of subjects had been wheeze-free for three or more years
- 27% experienced symptoms at least once a week
- the remaining 41% had less frequent wheezing episodes
- 27% who had minimal symptoms at the age of 14 had suffered from significant wheezing by the age of 21 years, and similarly at 28 years[46].

Asthma in teenagers: It has been suggested that severity of symptoms decreases in teenage years. However, recent studies suggest that the prevalence of asthma is as common in adolescence as it is in younger children[47] (Table 2.3).

Similar studies are not yet available for the UK. However, this research suggests that asthma may be underdiagnosed in teenagers.

Table 2.3 Prevalence of wheezing/asthma in adolescence

Country	Year	Age	Selection criteria	Prevalence (%)	Ref
New Zealand	1991	12–15	Reported wheezing	32–38	48
Australia	1992	12–15	Diagnosed asthma	16.5	49
Netherlands	1989	10–23	Diagnosed asthma	19	50

Possible reasons for this are that:

■ the symptoms are less severe

■ they are better tolerated

■ there is a denial of symptoms in order to conform with peer pressures, or

■ teenagers are unwilling to seek advice from health professionals who may be seen as establishment figures.

It is likely that we will need to change our approach to the assessment and management of asthmatics in this age group, perhaps by the use of 'teenage support groups' which have proved useful in diabetes and asthma in America.

Asthma in the elderly: Epidemiological studies supported by respiratory function testing have demonstrated an asthma prevalence of 6.5% in patients over 65, 50% of whom were unknown to their GPs[51]. An American longitudinal study of patients diagnosed as asthmatics over the age of 60 showed that they had had symptoms and abnormal pulmonary function tests for a mean of 8.5 years before the diagnosis was made[52]. Many factors may contribute to the failure to make the diagnosis in this age group:

■ symptoms may be mistaken for cardiac disease or chronic obstructive pulmonary disease

■ many elderly patients have multi-organ disease

■ symptoms may be attributed to growing old, or

■ there may be a failing cognitive function.

Frequency of symptoms: Asthma affects different people in various ways and similarly, individuals respond differently to the wide variety of asthma medication available. Recently, Mullen did a cluster analysis on four studies[53-56] and suggested that asthmatic patients may be usefully classified according to four patterns of symptoms:

- infrequently
- mainly in the day time
- mainly in the night time
- continuously.

There are possible practical applications of this classification that includes a system of choosing treatment options according to the patient's symptom category. Future research will clarify whether this is in fact useful.

Seasonal factors: There are significant seasonal variations in asthma attacks that can be related to changes in exposure to different trigger factors (Figure 2.2). Tree pollens and oil-seed rape flowering produce an effect in the early spring, followed by grass pollens in summer and then a peak in moulds in the damp days of autumn. Viral infections tend to exacerbate asthma attacks during the winter months and in the weeks following school holidays when the children return to school[57].

While the house dust mite has a perennial effect, there are peaks in early winter when central heating systems are switched on.

Morbidity

Uncontrolled asthma, whether acute or chronic, interferes with the patient's ability to function normally. Activities such as carrying the washing from the top flat to the drying green, taking the push-chair up one flight of stairs or cutting the grass become an effort. Disturbed sleep may reduce school performance[3]. A cold may cause chest symptoms lasting 2–3 weeks with time lost off school or work. Severe chronic asthma, even when treated with modern medicines, may lead to significant structural damage and a degree of permanent disability which cannot be reversed.

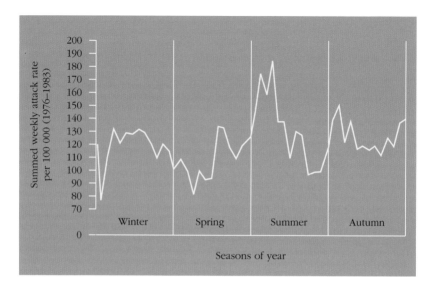

Figure 2.2 *Seasonal variations in asthma attacks. (Modified from Ayres JG[101])*

Nocturnal symptoms in 30–40% of asthmatic patients have been found in some studies[58,59]. A recent national audit of 6732 asthmatic patients registered with 225 GPs throughout the UK revealed that 58% had reported symptoms at their last assessment: 12% had taken time off work or school in the previous month, 24% had had an acute episode and 19% had been prescribed a course of steroids in the past year[60].

Simple measures of lung function may provide additional objective information on the morbidity suffered by people with asthma. For example, patients may deny having symptoms while peak flow measurements reveal significant variability or be unable to detect episodes of deterioration of peak expiratory flow[61].

The number of days lost off school, work or from household duties is a useful indicator of how asthma interferes with everyday life. Official figures show a rise in days of certified incapacity due to asthma from just under 4 million in 1977/80 to 10.5 million in 1991/92 in spite of changes in reporting of absences during this time. A similar rise has been seen in those claiming Invalidity Benefit due to asthma[42].

The numbers of patients consulting for asthma episodes has increased exponentially over the last decade (Figure 2.3). The weekly return service of the Royal College of General Practitioners provided data indicating a mean annual GP consultation rate for asthma episodes of 18.3 per 1000 population for males and 16.6 for females. The majority of these consultations were for children under four years old[44].

Hospital admissions for childhood asthma have more than doubled since the mid-1970s. A repeated yearly pattern of admissions was recognized in a study of 11 years' admissions to a children's hospital and this was attributed to a largely viral aetiology for asthmatic attacks throughout the year. The authors postulated that school holidays disrupt the spread of viral infections in a community, with synchronization of subsequent attacks[57]. Other researchers on hospital admissions have noted a seasonal variation being lowest in January–March with peaks in April, May, August/September, and October/November that are believed to be related to different allergens (Figure 2.4)[62,63].

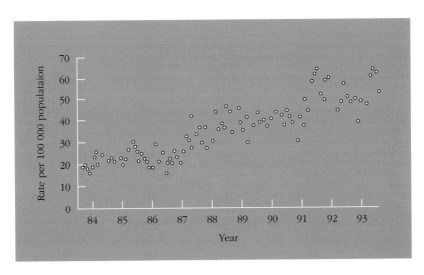

Figure 2.3 *Increasing workload in general practice. Mean weekly incidence of asthma consultations 1984 to 1993. The numbers of patients consulting for asthma episodes has increased exponentially over the last decade. (Source: RCGP Birmingham Research Unit, with permission.)*

19

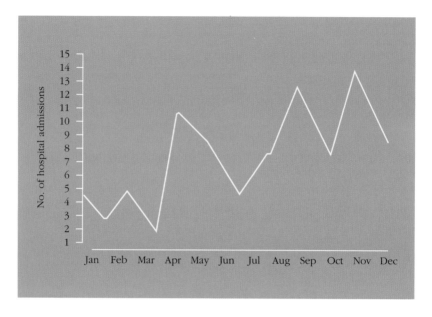

Figure 2.4 *Patterns of hospital admissions throughout the year. Comparison with Khot et al[100].*

There are problems related to the care of patients with asthma from different ethnic groups in the UK. A thorough understanding of cultural issues and access to interpreters may be of help in planning treatment and health gain issues[64,65]. Poor communication between health professionals and patients as well as cultural problems and compliance with drug therapy are thought to play a part in this morbidity[66].

Mortality

The death rate for asthma is relatively low when compared with chronic obstructive airways disease, bronchitis and bronchopneumonia. Asthma deaths relate more to older patients and, in many cases, are considered preventable[67–72].

Table 2.4 shows selected annual death rates for asthma since 1969. Asthma deaths increased in the late 1960s from the overuse of non-specific beta-agonist inhalers and underuse of corticosteroids in the management of acute attack. There was a steady increase in overall death rates during the 1970s and 1980s but this has fallen by 10% in the early 1990s. The major increase was in the over-65 age group which may reflect changes in diagnosis and classification rather than a real increase. Since 1969 there has been a steady fall in the number of deaths in the 0–14 age group[42]. However, mortality from asthma in the 10–20-year age group in the UK for 1990–1992 differs from other age groups. The death rate in this group has not declined and there is a preponderance in males[47,73].

A series of studies looking at asthma deaths both within the community and in the hospital setting has suggested that there are potentially preventable factors in up to 85% of cases. That is not to say that deaths would not have occurred, but it highlights the areas where management could be improved. Poor patient education is a recurring theme in these studies. The introduction of self-management plans, including home peak flow meters, have enabled patients to take more control of their asthma management with some success[74–85]. However, the most vulnerable patients are often the least compliant.

Table 2.4 Selected annual number of deaths from asthma for England 1969–92

Age (years)	1969	1975	1980	1985	1989	1992
0–4	26	16	11	12	6	10
5–14	38	20	27	19	13	8
15–44	222	174	181	260	225	167
45–64	473	367	431	574	448	385
65+	484	510	722	974	1109	1085
Total						
All ages	1243	1087	1372	1839	1801	1655
<65	759	577	650	865	692	570

Source: *Morbidity Statistics from General Practice 1991/92*, 1995.
Crown copyright 1995. Reproduced by permission of the Controller of HMSO and the Office for National Statistics.

Patients, relatives and doctors tend to underestimate the severity of an asthma attack and the speed with which deterioration can occur[67,69–71,86]. Evidence suggests that while improvements have taken place in the past decade there is no room for complacency and efforts need to be redoubled if we are to reduce the number of preventable deaths.

Where is asthma treated?

The day-to-day management of asthma has always been largely in the hands of GPs with a maximum of 5% of cases attending a hospital out-patient clinic at any one time. In a well resourced practice asthma clinic, this percentage is usually between 1% and 2%, with few adults and children over the age of 4 being referred. Community-based care is preferable to repeated visits to an out-patient clinic which may be staffed by a relatively inexperienced senior house officer rotating every 3–6 months.

However, in the inner city and deprived areas where the community services are overstretched, or from practices with little interest in asthma, the hospital services may take a larger share of the load. There are some areas where the expertise of the hospital service may be of particular value. Children under the age of 2 form a difficult group and until more is known about the natural history and response to treatment in this age group such referrals would seem appropriate. In the elderly, more sophisticated respiratory function tests may help to distinguish between asthma and chronic obstructive pulmonary disease. Other situations where hospital referral might be appropriate are discussed in Chapter 7; however, once the patient has been assessed by the hospital most cases can be discharged back to the care of the GP.

Patients recently discharged from hospital need proper assessment and follow-up to prevent relapse. Whether this is best done in the hospital respiratory clinic or a GP asthma clinic depends on the facilities available in each individual case.

While hospital admissions for childhood asthma may have doubled over the last 20 years, the length of stay has fallen. It was initially thought that this change was due to increased morbidity alone. However, changing trends in the provision and use of the National Health Service, with the introduction of direct-access admissions and lack of out-of-hours community cover in inner cities, means that hospitals provide a consultation service in these areas[63].

A national audit of the management of acute asthma attacks in the community involving 218 practices from throughout the UK and collecting information on 1805 acute attacks, showed 95% of acute episodes were seen initially by the GP and 86% were managed wholly within the community. In this study only 5% self-referred to an A&E department[88]. However, there is audit evidence that suggests that in some areas, a higher proportion of patients self-refer to the A&E departments[79,89].

In a prospective controlled study[90] of 145 children with asthma, classified as 'repeated attenders' in a Liverpool A&E department, 81% were self-referred. The study concluded that the symptoms of those attending A&E repeatedly (n = 145) were more severe than the controls (n = 118). The major determinant of attendance was the parent's conviction that appropriate treatment could not be obtained elsewhere.

The age distribution of the 12% of the cases admitted to hospital in the national audit[88] of acute attacks is shown in Table 2.5. Three-quarters of those under the age of 4 were males and most admissions were under the age of 19. Of interest is the number of women aged 20–39 — this coincides with the child-bearing age when mothers often take less care of their own health and more concern over their offspring. These findings have been confirmed by other studies.

An audit of the management of acute asthma within hospitals from the Glasgow area showed that care was significantly better if undertaken by respiratory rather than general physicians. As a result

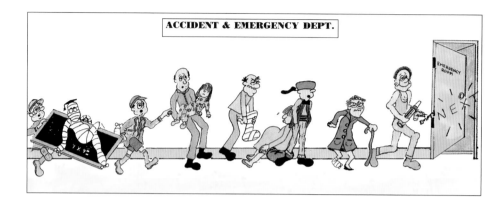

Table 2.5 Age distribution of numbers of patients admitted in the National Audit[88]

Sex	Age (years)							
	0–9	10–19	20–29	30–39	40–49	50–59	60–69	≥70
Male	47	12	6	4	2	4	4	8
Female	19	9	13	6	5	0	6	10

of an educational programme a re-audit of the same hospital showed considerable improvement in management by general physicians[91–93].

The health economics of asthma

There is an ever increasing demand on the health-care services. People's expectations are rising as are the costs of providing the service. However, the budgets available are limited. Choices have to be made, but health-care professionals find such choices difficult. Between 1 and 2% of the total medical budget in developed countries goes on asthma care and there is evidence that these costs are increasing faster than for the other health sectors. Is the current budget for asthma care being appropriately used or can improvements be achieved within that budget?

When the cost implications of asthma and its management are considered, it soon becomes clear that different sectors of the service are contributing to the overall picture. Problems arise when each sector looks only at its own cost without considering the implications to the service as a whole. For instance, the Health Boards or Health Authorities may look at the rising costs of prophylactic medication without considering the reduction in out-of-hours calls, hospital out-patient and in-patient referrals and reduced sickness payments.

A study from East London found that prescription costs for asthma were higher in a training practice which following approved guidelines[94]. However, a strict application of management guidelines has been shown to reduce both morbidity and the need for hospitalization[95,96]. Work from Sweden has shown that areas of the country with a high prescription rate of inhaled steroids had the lowest admission rates for asthma[97]. It has been estimated that one hospital admission for asthma is equal to several years' worth of inhaled steroids for that patient.

Overall management costs will depend on the severity of asthma; the most severe 10% of asthmatics consume over 50% of the total drug costs for asthma and a significant percentage of the overall health-care costs, including hospitalization[98].

When mild-to-moderate asthma is considered, where drugs account for 85% of the costs, a reduction in hospitalization is a less useful parameter as these patients are rarely admitted. In these circumstances, outcome measures such as the quality of life, symptom-free days or a reduction in the number of exacerbations, take on greater importance. In this respect, a recent study comparing two inhaled steroids showed that while both appeared to be as efficacious in controlling lung function, one was considerably superior in reducing the number of exacerbations[55]. More studies of this type are needed if our prescribing is to become more cost effective.

The establishment of a resourced asthma clinic invariably leads to an increase in prescription costs. Results from one such practice showed an increase in prescription costs from £39 706 in 1987/88 to £89 040 in 1993/94 largely as the result of a rise in spending on inhaled corticosteroids from £14 374 to £53 640[99]. However, during this period the number of registered asthmatics in the practice increased from 345 to 1106 due to an increase in the number being diagnosed, an increase in the practice size and evidence that asthmatic patients were actively joining the practice. The number of patients receiving inhaled steroids rose from 110 to 694 but the average prescription costs per asthmatic fell from £115 to £80. This illustrates how complicated the calculations can become and the difficulties that may be encountered if global figures are taken at face value.

Efforts are now being made to try to provide realistic costings for the various items of asthma service. This is a very complex process but Neville *et al.* suggested a methodology for looking at overall costs of providing asthma care in children[87]. Figures will vary from area to area depending on the level and organization within individual practices, the staffing levels and availability of high tech equipment within the local district general hospital, costs per day of admission being much higher in teaching hospitals. Clearly it is much cheaper to see patients in a well resourced, nurse-led practice asthma clinic, than for the patient to be followed up in a hospital out-patient department. Many fund-holding practices are aware of these facts and are now asking for assessment and return when referring patients to hospital clinics.

Costings are usually based on the cheapest effective treatments, which may well mean the use of a generic steroid pressurized metered-dose inhaler via a spacer device, and take little account of the more sophisticated devices often needed to manage childhood asthma.

The Facilitator study[87] involving 12 representative Tayside general practices showed an initial rise in practice-initiated reviews during the second year from 413 to 902 but a fall to 330 by the fourth year. There was also a fall in non-asthma respiratory consultations from 1720 in year one to 368 in year four. Overall general practitioner respiratory consultations including asthma fell from 2518 to 1160 with an estimated reduction in costs from £22 980 to £10 170. The costs of maintenance therapy had, however, risen from £19 830 to £24 680, but against this must be set a fall in hospital admissions from 50 in the first year to 14 in year four, giving a reduction in in-patient costs from £20 430 to £5720. With all factors taken into account it was estimated that the setting up of an effective asthma screening programme for children with asthma-like symptoms reduced the yearly costs after four years from £68 499 to £43 554 (37%). However, these rather crude figures hide a 22% fall in the number of children taking treatment, i.e. those who had 'grown out' of their asthma. In adults one would also have to take into account savings from the reduction in sickness benefit and loss of taxes.

In this chapter we have presented a brief summary of several different topics relating to asthma which may help health-care professionals to understand the disease better and aid them when they are considering management options. From the evidence presented it is clear that while enormous strides have been made, particularly in the last 10 years, a lot of work still needs to be done. Primary care has accepted its key role in the management of asthma and is organizing itself into an effective force to achieve these objectives.

References

1 Costa Pereira ANR. *Asthma-like symptoms in the community: a study of care.* PhD Thesis Dundee University, 1993.

2 Lenney W, Wells NEJ, O'Neill BA. The burden of paediatric asthma. *Eur Resp Rev* 1994; **4**: 49–62.

3 Action Asthma. *Young Asthmatics Survey*, 1993, Uxbridge, Middlesex, UK.

4 Donnelly JE, Donnelly WJ, Thong YH. Parental perceptions and attitudes toward asthma and its treatment: a controlled study. *Social Sci Med* 1987; **24**: 431–7.

5 Coughlin SP. Sport and the asthmatic child: a study of exercise induced asthma and resultant handicap. *J Roy Coll Gen Pract* 1988; **38**: 253–5.

6 Nocon A, Booth T. The social impact of asthma. *Fam Pract* 1991; **8**: 37–41.

7 Anon. *The occurrence and cost of asthma.* Cambridge: Cambridge Medical Publications, 1990.

8 British Lung Foundation. *The Lung report. Lung disease: a shadow over the nation's health.* 1996; 1–40.

9 Scottish Health Service. *Scottish Health Statistics.* Common Service Agency, Divisions 1 and 5. Edinburgh: HMSO, 1990.

10 Royal College of General Practitioners/Office of Population Censuses and Surveys, Department of Health and Social Security. *Morbidity statistics from general practice 1981–82. Third national study.* London: HMSO, 1986.

11 Slater HH. *On asthma: its pathology and treatment.* London: Churchill, 1986.

12 CIBA Foundation Guest Symposium: Terminology, definitions and classifications of chronic pulmonary emphysema and related conditions. *Thorax* 1959; 14–286.

13 American Thoracic Society. Chronic bronchitis, asthma and pulmonary emphysema. A Statement by a Committee on diagnostic standard for non-tuberculous respiratory disease. *Am Rev Resp Dis* 1962; **85**: 762–8.

14 Scadding JC. Definition and clinical categories of asthma. In: Clark TJH and Godfrey S, eds. *Asthma.* London: Chapman and Hall, 1983.

15 Global Initiative for Asthma. *Global strategy for asthma management and prevention.* NHLBI/WHO workshop report. NIH publication no. 95–3659, 1995: 1–46.

16 Strachan DP. Epidemiology. In: Silverman M, ed. *Childhood asthma and other wheezing disorders.* London: Chapman Hall, 1995; 7–31.

17 Burrows B, Lebowitz MD, Barbee RA. Respiratory disorders and allergy skin-test reactions. *Ann Intern Med* 1976; **84**: 134–9.

18 Platts-Mills TA, Ward GW Jr, Sporik R, Gelber LE, Chapman MD, Heymann PW. Epidemiology of the relationship between exposure to indoor allergens and asthma. *Int Arch Allergy Appl Immunol* 1991; **94**: 339–45.

19 Sporik R, Holgate ST, Platts-Mills TA, Cogswell JJ. Exposure to house-dust mite allergen and the development of asthma in childhood. A prospective study. *New Engl J Med* 1990; **323**: 502–7.

20 Hide DW, Matthews S, Matthews L *et al.* Effect of allergen avoidance in infancy on allergic manifestations at age two years. *J Allergy Clin Immunol* 1994; **93**: 842–6.

21 Royal College of Physicians. *Smoking and the Young.* 1992; 1–23.

22 Godfrey KM *et al.* Disproportionate foetal growth and raised IgE concentrations in adult life. *Clin Exp Allergy* 1996; **24**: 641–8.

23 Burney PGJ. Epidemiology. In: Clark TJH, Godfrey S, Lee TH, eds. *Asthma.* London, New York, Tokyo, Melbourne, Madras: Chapman & Hall, 1992; 254–307.

24 Anto JM, Sunyer J, Rodriguez-Roisin R, Suarez-Cervera M, Vazquez L. Community outbreaks of asthma associated with inhalation of soybean dust. *New Engl J Med* 1989; **320**: 1097–102.

25 Celenza A, Fothergill J, Shaw RJ. Thunderstorm associated asthma: a detailed analysis of environmental factors. *BMJ* 1996; **312**: 604–7.

26 Davidson AC, Emberlin J, Cook AD, Venables KM. A major outbreak of asthma associated with a thunderstorm: experience of accident and emergency departments and patients' characteristics. *BMJ* 1996; **312**: 601–4.

27 Bellomo R, Gigliotti P, Treolar A *et al.* Two consecutive thunderstorm associated epidemics of asthma in the city of Melbourne. The possible role of rye grass pollen. *Med J Austral* 1992; **157**: 352–3.

28 Packe GE, Ayres JG. Asthma outbreak during a thunderstorm. *Lancet* 1985; **2**: 199–204.

29 Gellert AR, Gellert SL, Iliffe SR. Prevalence and management of asthma in a London inner city general practice. *Br J Gen Pract* 1990; **40**: 197–201.

30 Lee DA, Winslow NR, Speight AN, Hey EN. Prevalence and spectrum of asthma in childhood. *Br Med J Clin Res Ed* 1990; **286**: 1256–8.

31 Speight ANP, Lee DA, Hey EN. Underdiagnosis and undertreatment of asthma in childhood. *Br Med J Clin Res Ed* 1983; **286**: 1253–6.

32 Levy M, Bell L. General practice audit of asthma in childhood. *Br Med J* 1984: **289**: 1115–16.

33 Heeijne Den Bak J. Prevalence and management of asthma in children under 16 in one practice. *BMJ* 1986; **292**: 175–6.

34 Jones A, Sykes AP. The effect of symptom presentation on delay in asthma diagnosis in children in a general practice. *Resp Med* 1990; **84**: 139–42.

35 Anderson HR, Pottier AC, Strachan DP. Asthma from birth to age 23: incidence and relation to prior and concurrent atopic disease. *Thorax* 1992; **47**: 537–42.

36 Van Niekerk CH, Weinberg EG, Shore SC *et al.* Prevalence of asthma: a comparative study of urban and rural Xhosa children. *Clin Allergy* 1979; **9**: 319–24.

37 Godfrey RC. Asthma and IgE levels in rural and urban communities of The Gambia. *Clin Allergy* 1975; **5**: 201–7.

38 Anderson HR. Respiratory abnormalities in Papua New Guinea children — the effects of locality and domestic wood smoke. *Int J Epidemiol* 1978; **7**: 63.

39 Austin JB, Russell G, Adam MG, Mackintosh D, Kelsey S, Peck DF. Prevalence of asthma and wheeze in the highlands of Scotland. *Arch Dis Childhood* 1994; **71**: 211–16.

40 Bryce FP, Neville RG, Crombie IK, Clark RA, McKenzie P. Controlled trial of an audit facilitator in diagnosis and treatment of childhood asthma in general practice. *BMJ* 1995; **310**: 838–42.

41 Levy ML, Barnes GR, Howe M, Neville RG. Provision of primary care asthma services in the UK. *Thorax* 1996; **51**: A28.

42 Central Health Monitoring Unit. *Asthma. An epidemiological overview.* London: HMSO, 1995; 1–61.

43 Ninan TK, Russell G. Respiratory symptoms and atopy in Aberdeen school children: Evidence from two surveys 25 years apart. *BMJ* 1992; **304**: 873–5.

44 Office of Population Censuses and Surveys. *Morbidity statistics from general practice.* 1991/92 (MSGP4). OPCS Monitor 1994; MB5 94/1: 1–12.

45 Anderson HR, Bland JM, Patel S, Peckham C. The natural history of asthma in childhood. *J Epidemiol Commun Hlth* 1986; **40**: 121–9.

46 Kelly WJW, Hudson I, Phelan PD, Pain MCF, Olinsky A. Childhood asthma in adult life: a further study at 28 yrs of life. *BMJ* 1987; **294**: 1059–62.

47 Price JF. Issues of adolescent asthma: what are the needs? *Thorax* 1996; **51**: S1–S17.

48 Robson B, Woodman K, Burgess C, Crane J, Pearce N, Shaw R. Prevalence of asthma symptoms among adolescents in the Wellington region by area and ethnicity. *NZ Med J* 1993: **106**: 239–41.

49 Forero R, Bauman A, Young A, Larkin P. Asthma prevalence and management in Australian adolescents: results from three community surveys. *J Adolesc Hlth* 1992; **13**: 707–12.

50 Kolnaar B, Beissel E, van den Bosch WJ, Folgering H, van den Hoogen HJ, van Weel C. Asthma in adolescents and young adults: screening outcome versus diagnosis in general practice. *Fam Prac* 1994; **11**: 133–40.

51 Burr ML, Charles TJ, Roy K, Seaton A. Asthma in the elderly: an epidemiological survey. *BMJ* 1979; **1**: 1041–4.

52 Burrows B, Lebowitz MD, Barbee RA, Cline MG. Findings before diagnoses of asthma among the elderly in a longitudinal study of a general population sample. *J Allergy Clin Immunol* 1991; **88**: 870–7.

53 Britton MG, Earnshaw JS, Palmer JB. A twelve-month comparison of salmeterol with salbutamol in asthmatic patients. European Study Group. *Eur Resp J* 1992; **5**: 1062–7.

54 Greening AP, Ind PW, Northfield M, Shaw G. Added salmeterol versus higher-dose corticosteroid in asthma patients with symptoms on existing inhaled corticosteroid. Allen & Hanbury's Ltd UK Study Group. *Lancet* 1994; **344**: 219–24.

55 Fabbri L, Burge PS, Croonenborgh L *et al.* Comparison of fluticasone propionate with beclomethasone dipropionate in moderate to severe asthma treated for one year. International Study Group. *Thorax* 1993; **48**: 817–23.

56 Woolcock A, Lundback B, Ringdal N, Jacques LA. Comparison of addition of salmeterol to inhaled steroids with doubling of the dose of inhaled steroids. *Am J Resp Crit Care Med* 1996; **153**: 1481–8.

57 Storr J, Lenney W. School holidays and admissions with asthma. *Arch Disease Childhood* 1989; **64**: 103–7.

58 White PT, Pharoah CA, Anderson HR, Freeling P. Randomized controlled trial of small group education on the outcome of chronic asthma in general practice. *J Roy Coll Gen Pract* 1989; **39**: 182–6.

59 Turner-Warwick M. Nocturnal asthma: a study in general practice. *J Roy Coll Gen Pract* 1989; **39**: 239–43.

60 Neville RG, Hoskins G, Smith B, Clark RA. Observations on the structure, process and clinical outcomes of asthma care in general practice. *Br J Gen Pract* 1996; **46**: 583–7.

61 Kendrick AH, Higgs CM, Whitfield MJ, Laszlo G. Accuracy of perception of severity of asthma: patients treated in general practice. *BMJ* 1993; **307**: 422–4.

62 Anderson HR. Increase in hospital admissions for childhood asthma: trends in referral, severity, and readmissions from 1970 to 1985 in a health region of the UK. *Thorax* 1989; **44**: 614–19.

63 Strachan DP, Anderson HR. Trends in hospital admission rates for asthma in children. *BMJ* 1992; **304**: 819–20.

64 MacFadyen UM, Aslam M, McCarthy TP, Patel J, Lakhani N. A study of cultural issues relating to asthma and its management among Asian patients. *Thorax* 1996; **51**: A30(Abs).

65 Mougdil H, Honeybourne D. Differences in asthma management between white European and Indian subcontinent groups. *Thorax* 1996; **51**: A30(Abs).

66 Ayres JG. Acute asthma in Asian patients, hospital admissions and duration of stay in a district with a high immigrant population. *Br J Dis Chest* 1986; **92**: 42.

67 Eason J, Markowe HJL. Controlled investigation of deaths from asthma in hospitals in the North-East Thames region. *BMJ* 1987; **294**: 1255–8.

68 Asthma mortality task force (1986). American Academy of Allergy and Immunology and the American Thoracic Society. *J Allergy Clin Immunol* 1987; **80**: 361–514.

69 Wright SC, Evans AE, Sinnamon DG, MacMahon J. Asthma mortality and death certification in Northern Ireland. *Thorax* 1994; **49**: 141–3.

70 British Thoracic Association. Death from asthma in two regions. *BMJ* 1982; **285**: 1251–5.

71 Wareham NJ, Harrison BD, Jenkins PF, Nicholls J, Stableforth DE. A district confidential enquiry into deaths due to asthma. *Thorax* 1993; **48**: 1117–20.

72 The British Thoracic Society, The National Asthma Campaign, The Royal College of Physicians of London *et al.* British Guidelines on Asthma Management: 1995. Review and Position Statement. *Thorax* 1997; 52 (Suppl. 1): S1–S21.

73 OPCS. *Office of Population and Census Surveys DH 2.* 1996.

74 Hayward SA, Jordan M, Golden G, Levy M. A randomised controlled evaluation of asthma self management in general practice. *Asthma Gen Pract* 1996; **4**: 11–13.

75 Lahdensuo A, Haahtela T, Herrala J *et al.* Randomised comparison of guided self management and traditional treatment of asthma over one year. *BMJ* 1996; **312**: 748–52.

76 Brewin AM, Hughes JA. Effect of patient education on asthma management. *Br J Nurs* 1995; **4**: 81–2.

77 D'Souza W, Crane J, Beasley R. Self-management plans. In: O'Byrne PO, Thomson NC, eds. *Manual of asthma management.* London, Philadelphia, Toronto, Sydney, Tokyo: W.B. Saunders Company Ltd, 1995; 393–412.

78 Ignacio-Garcia JM, Gonzalez-Santos P. Asthma self-management education program by home monitoring of peak expiratory flow. *Am J Resp Crit Care Med* 1995; **151**: 353–9.

79 Levy ML, Robb M, Allen J, Doherty C, Bland M, Winter RJD. Guided self-management reduces morbidity, time off work and consultations for uncontrolled asthma in adults. *Eur Resp J* 1995; Supplement 19: 318s(Abs).

80 Partridge MR. Delivering optimal care to the person with asthma: what are the key components and what do we mean by patient education? *Eur Resp J* 1995; **8**: 298–305.

81 Charlton I, Antoniou AG, Atkinson J *et al.* Asthma at the interface: bridging the gap between general practice and a district general hospital. *Arch Dis Childhood* 1994; **70**: 313–18.

82 D'Souza W, Crane J, Burgess C *et al.* Community-based asthma care: trial of a "credit card" asthma self-management plan. *Eur Resp J* 1994; **7**: 1260–5.

83 Brewis RA. Patient education, self–management plans and peak flow measurement [Review]. *Resp Med* 1991; **85**: 457–62.

84 Charlton I, Charlton G. New perspectives in asthma self-management. *Practitioner* 1990; **234**: 30–32.

85 Beasley R, Cushley M, Holgate ST. A self management plan in the treatment of adult asthma. *Thorax* 1989; **44**: 200–4.

86 Fletcher HJ, Ibrahim SA, Speight N. Survey of asthma deaths in the Northern region, 1970–85. *Arch Dis Childhood* 1990; **65**: 163–7.

87 McCowan C, Neville RG, Crombie IK, Clark RA, Warner FC. The facilitator effect: results from a 4-year follow-up of children with asthma. *Br J Gen Pract* 1997; **47**: 156–60.

88 Neville RG, Clark RC, Hoskins G, Smith B. National asthma attack audit 1991–2. General Practitioners in Asthma Group. *BMJ* 1993; **306**: 559–62.

89 Levy ML, Robb M, Bradley JL, Winter RJD. Presentation and self management in acute asthma: a prospective study in two districts. *Thorax* 1993; **48**: 460–1(Abs).

90 O'Halloran SM and Heaf DP. Recurrent accident and emergency department attendance for acute asthma in children. *Thorax* 1989; **44**: 620–6.

91 Bucknall CE, Robertson C, Moran F, Stevenson RD. Improving management of asthma: closing the loop or progressing along the audit spiral? *Quality Hlth Care* 1992; **1**: 15–20.

92 Bucknall CE, Robertson C, Moran F, Stevenson RD. Management of asthma in hospital: a prospective audit. *BMJ* 1988; **296**: 1637–9.

93 Bucknall CE, Robertson C, Moran F, Stevenson RD. Differences in hospital asthma management. *Lancet* 1988; **1**: 748–50.

94 Naish J, Sturdy P, Toon P. Appropriate prescribing in asthma and its related cost in east London. *BMJ* 1995; **310**: 97–100.

95 Charlton I, Charlton G, Broomfield J, Mullee MA. Evaluation of peak flow and symptoms only self management plans for control of asthma in general practice [see comments]. *BMJ* 1990; **301**: 1355–9.

96 Trautner C, Richter B, Berger M. Cost-effectiveness of a structured treatment and teaching programme on asthma. *Eur Respir J* 1993; **6**: 1485–91.

97 Gerdtham UG, Hertzman P, Jonsson B, Boman G. Impact of inhaled corticosteroids on the asthma population in Sweden: a pooled regression analysis. Research report of the Bkomomiska Forsking Institutet, Centre for Health Economics, Stockholm, 1995.

98 Scheffer A. *Global strategy for asthma management and prevention.* NHLBI/WHO Workshop Report. 1995; 95–3659: 1–176.

99 Price DB. Inhaled steroid prescribing over seven years in a general practice and its implications. *Eur Resp J* 1995; Supplement 19: 463s.

100 Khot A, Evans N, Lenney W. Seasonal trends in childhood asthma in South East England. *BMJ* 1983; **287**: 1257–8.

101 Ayres JG. Trends in asthma and hay fever in general practice in the United Kingdom 1976–83. *Thorax* 1986; **41**: 111–16.

Chapter 3

Pathogenesis and molecular mechanisms

Henry Hyde Salter, a physician from Charing Cross Hospital in London, had first described the clinical basis of asthma as 'periodic paroxysmal dyspnoea' in 1868[1], although it was William Osler (1892) who alluded to the importance of airway inflammation by describing asthma as 'a special form of inflammation affecting the small bronchioles'[2]. Over 100 years on, asthma is now recognized as the most common treatable chronic disease of the lung afflicting all age groups, yet despite the new advances in treatment, particularly with more selective and potent drugs, there has been little impact on the rising morbidity and mortality from the disease. In the recognition that most asthma in childhood and young adults is associated with increased synthesis of IgE to common allergens or atopy, a better understanding of the pathophysiology of asthma has been gained from focusing on the role of airway inflammation, which in turn has offered new insights into how the disease may be treated[3].

Importance of airway inflammation in asthma

It has long been known that individuals dying from asthma have features of extensive airway inflammation with activation of airway mast cells and infiltration of the airway lumen with eosinophils, mononuclear cells and pro-inflammatory products. Despite this, it is surprising how little has been understood over the past 100 years about the pathogenesis and inflammatory events that occur within the airways of individuals suffering from day-to-day asthma, and how this relates to the clinical manifestation of the disease. The main reason for this has been the difficulty in gaining access to airway tissue in life. With the introduction of fibreoptic bronchoscopy and use of techniques such as bronchial biopsy and bronchoalveolar lavage (BAL), the last decade has seen a major change in how asthma is perceived as a disease of airway inflammation with functional consequences rather than solely in terms of disordered smooth muscle function[1]. Analyses of BAL fluid and biopsies have indicated that asthmatic airways, irrespective of disease severity, are involved in an inflammatory response involving eosinophils, mast cells and mononuclear cells, and that disordered airway function involves the secretion of stored and newly formed pro-inflammatory mediators.

National and international guidelines for the diagnosis and treatment of asthma have reflected the importance of these changes. In the recent Global Initiative for Asthma (GINA) in 1995 (a joint National Institutes for Health (NIH) and World Health Organization (WHO) project)[5], two forms of asthma have been recognized:

■ an intermittent form involving exacerbations of symptoms separated by weeks or months of normal lung function and absence of symptoms, and

■ a persistent form which can range from mild to severe.

These forms are the two ends of a spectrum, and common to both is the presence of 'chronic inflammation of the airways in which many cells play a role, in particular mast cells, eosinophils and T lymphocytes, that cause recurrent episodes of wheezing, chest tightness and cough in susceptible individuals.' The latter statement is now an important component of the WHO definition of asthma.

Airway hyperresponsiveness (twitchiness) and airway obstruction are the two principal consequences of airway inflammation.

Bronchial hyperresponsiveness

An abnormal state of airway function referred to as bronchial hyperresponsiveness (BHR) is provoked by a wide range of internal and external stimuli. The state of BHR describing the magnitude of airway narrowing is often called 'non-specific' although, in practice, the stimuli act by highly specific mechanisms. They may be classified as those causing airway obstruction:

■ directly by stimulating airway smooth muscle, such as inhaled methacholine and histamine, or

■ indirectly by releasing pharmacologically active mediators from secreting cells such as mast cells (e.g. exercise) or sensory neurones (e.g. sulphur dioxide) (Figure 3.1).

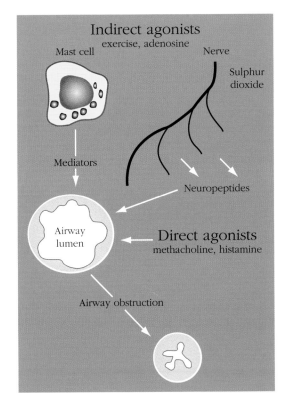

Figure 3.1 *The concept of direct and indirect bronchial hyperresponsiveness.*

35

In the laboratory, controlled stimulation of the airway enables the quantification of BHR by analysis of dose-response curves. By plotting the shape and position of the curve, the dose or concentration of agonist required to provoke a specified fall in lung function (usually forced expiratory volume in one second — FEV_1) can be determined. This method of measurement of BHR has been standardized for methacholine and histamine, and the provocative dose (or concentration) that reduces FEV_1 by 20% is used most commonly (PD_{20} or PC_{20})[6] (Figure 3.2).

When responsiveness is normal, the dose–response curve is displaced to the right, indicating that a high dose is required to cause airway constriction, and there is also a maximal response plateau. When BHR is enhanced, the curve is shifted to the left and the maximal response plateau is increased and eventually lost. Care is required in the interpretation of the curves: the cut-off point between normal and increased BHR is dependent on the agonist used, and the population studied. For example, the relationship between FEV_1 and BHR to methacholine is different between cigarette smokers and non-smokers[7].

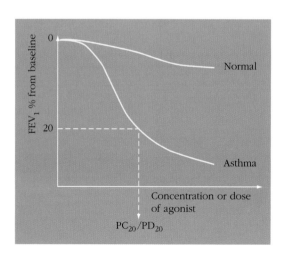

Figure 3.2 *Dose–response relationship between bronchoconstrictor agonist and reduction in normal and asthmatic airway calibre.*

BHR testing as a diagnostic tool

BHR tests have an important diagnostic role in individuals suspected of having asthma, although they have to be interpreted judiciously, especially in children[8]. Measurement of airway responsiveness to histamine or methacholine is useful in patients in whom the diagnosis of asthma is uncertain but who present with typical symptoms and normal spirometry. In such instances, the presence of BHR suggests that the symptoms are associated with asthma, and the absence of BHR suggests that asthma is not present, although it does not exclude it. Many of the reasons for the poor relationship between the degree of airway responsiveness, symptoms and asthma have stemmed from epidemiological studies showing that many people are hyperresponsive but have no symptoms, whilst others with symptoms or a previous diagnosis of asthma have normal airway responsiveness[9–11]. Although BHR without symptoms may be due to a failure to recognize symptoms or variable airway obstruction[12,13], it is the presence of symptoms in the absence of BHR that is more difficult to explain. Possible explanations include the presence of:

- responsiveness in the normal or 'borderline' range associated with symptoms,
- other bronchoconstrictor stimuli that are not reflected by the agonist used in the provocation tests, e.g. stimuli from occupational exposures[14].

Despite these caveats, BHR testing is an important diagnostic tool, and has advantages over other methods used to 'test' for asthma. They have particular advantages over 'bronchodilator tests' for asthma which are based on the concept of increased basal airway tone. The bronchodilator method of demonstrating 'reversibility', which involves measuring a 15–20% change in lung function (FEV_1 or PEF) after inhalation of a beta-2 agonist, is of diagnostic help only if the baseline index of lung function is $\leq 80\%$ of the predicted value. In those individuals with a greatly reduced baseline airway function, or those with a baseline airway calibre that falls within the normal range, it is important to consider the absolute changes in lung volume rather than rely solely on percentage changes in function. It is in the latter circumstance that BHR testing is particularly useful.

The clinical consequences of enhanced BHR is often reflected in the increased variability in airway calibre and function both within and between days; the diurnal variation in peak expiratory flow (PEF) which correlates well with FEV_1, is highly characteristic of asthma and correlates well with responsiveness to histamine or methacholine[15]. When BHR is increased, diurnal variation in PEF is also increased, often even when there are no symptoms. Whilst the strength of the relationship of BHR to PEF is useful clinically, it should not detract from the importance of BHR testing, particularly because BHR tests are more accurate, sensitive and reproducible, and results can often be obtained more quickly in suitably equipped laboratories.

Airway obstruction

Perhaps of most concern to the clinician are the prolonged episodes of airway obstruction, with or without increases in airway responsiveness, which punctuate the life of patients with asthma, and still remain the most frequent reason for the patient to consult the practitioner. The recurrent episodes of airway obstruction in asthmatic individuals are usually a result of allergen-provoked airway inflammation and the functional consequence of airway obstruction.

Early and late bronchoconstriction

The mechanisms of acute bronchoconstriction varies according to the stimulus. The sensitized airways of asthmatic patients respond to inhaled allergen by producing an acute phase of bronchoconstriction, or the early asthmatic response (EAR). The EAR reaches a maximum 15–20 minutes after challenge and recovers over the following hour. This is followed by a late asthmatic response (LAR) starting at around 2–4 hours, reaching a maximum at 6–8 hours, followed by recovery usually over 24 hours. These events are paralleled by an increase in acquired BHR (to agents such as methacholine and histamine) that can persist for several days after the resolution of the LAR. The reduction in airway calibre during the EAR is rapidly reversed by beta-2 agonists. Whilst corticosteroids inhibit the LAR and acquired BHR, nedocromil sodium and sodium cromoglycate inhibit all three components[16]. The measurement of mediators in the peripheral circulation, bronchoalveolar lavage (BAL) and urine have confirmed that the release of inflammatory mediators from mast cells are important in the EAR after allergen challenge. More convincing evidence has come from studies using specific mediators such as histamine (HT)-1, leukotriene (LT)D4, prostaglandin (PG)D2 and thromboxane (TX)A2 receptor antagonists[17–19], and 5-lipoxygenase and cyclo-oxygenase inhibitors[20,21] which show attenuation of the EAR after allergen provocation[18]. The mediators most likely to account for the acute bronchoconstriction in these reactions are LTC4, PGD2 (and its metabolite $9\alpha,11\beta$-PGF2)[22] and histamine in descending order of potency. The rapid bronchoconstriction is due to contraction of the airway smooth muscle which contains receptors for mast cell-derived histamine, LTC4, LTD4, TXA2 and PGD2. The cellular biology of the LAR will be discussed later in the chapter.

Airway wall swelling and remodelling

There are other changes in airway structure, particularly of the airway wall, that contribute to airway obstruction in asthma. The epithelium in the airway wall is disrupted and often absent, and if present contains an excess of goblet and squamous cells. The basement membrane is markedly thickened owing to a band of subepithelial fibrosis that contains an excess of Type I, III and V collagen[23], probably deposited by myofibroblast cells whose number and activity increase in asthma[24]. The airway wall is also thickened because of an inflammatory exudate and increase (hyperplasia) in airway smooth muscle[25]. Elements of submucosal connective tissue other than muscle are also increased, accompanied by an expansion of the microvascular space that also contributes to the swelling in the airway wall. The structural changes are therefore consistent with a chronic inflammatory process with two distinct features:

■ one involves the mucus-secreting surface whereby the goblet cells and bronchial glands empty in response to irritants, and

■ the other involves epithelial disruption with shedding.

Although the mechanisms for the latter are not known, it may either be:

■ a cytolytic response to potent eosinophil-derived products, particularly major basic protein[26]

■ a mechanical consequence of increased pressure in the submucosa related to smooth muscle shortening, or

■ as recently suggested, a result of damage to the intraepithelial adhesive mechanisms by proteolytic enzymes derived from eosinophils or epithelial cells[27].

More recent evidence has suggested a role for growth factors expressed by inflammatory cells as a potent stimulus for tissue growth evident in asthmatic airways. In particular, the ability of interleukin (IL)-4[28], tumour necrosis factor (TNF)-α[29], platelet-derived growth factor (PDGF), endothelin-1 and transforming growth factor (TGF)-β_1[30] to induce fibrogenic responses has received attention, because this implies that permanent lung damage may ensue.

The main functional consequences of these structural changes are an increase in airway obstruction (with consequent rises in airway resistance) and bronchial hyperresponsiveness. There is evidence, based on computer simulation models, suggesting that a given amount of smooth muscle shortening will cause greater narrowing of the airway lumen when the airway wall is thickened compared to when it is normal[31]. Perhaps of more importance is the evidence showing where the structural changes in asthma have their greatest effect. Again, based on computer modelling, if asthmatic changes are present throughout the airways, airway resistance rises progressively. If, however, the changes are limited to the peripheral airways, then these airways will close with even modest amounts of smooth muscle shortening, and the airway resistance will be similar to that when all the airways are affected[32]. This indicates that asthmatic changes in the smaller airways, where smooth muscle completely encircles the lumen, may be more important than previously recognized; although, of course, acute narrowing of central airways has a disproportionate effect on increasing total airway resistance and therefore increasing the work of breathing during a severe asthma attack.

Changes in airway permeability are closely mirrored by changes in airway hyperresponsiveness following an acute or subacute inflammatory reaction. This can be explained by exposure of sensory nerve endings to toxic stimuli. The airway responsiveness of chronic asthma is more difficult to explain, particularly since it has been difficult to demonstrate increases in permeability even in patients with severe disease; there is some evidence that this may be related to increased wall thickness as a result of the inflammatory process.

The changes described above indicate that the increased airway obstruction and hyperresponsiveness characteristic of asthma can be explained by the combination of airway wall thickening which acts in series with smooth muscle shortening, both of which are a result of the chronic inflammatory process. The clinical relevance is that even in the absence of symptoms, overt airway obstruction or hyperresponsiveness, asthma will still manifest in the form of airway inflammation of variable degree, and is perhaps the most important variable factor determining the severity of clinical asthma.

Airway inflammation

The previous account has described the current concept of asthma as a chronic inflammatory process involving the airway wall resulting in airway obstruction and hyperresponsiveness, thus predisposing the airways to constrict to a variety of stimuli (Figure 3.3).

This inflammatory response is specifically characterized by the airway infiltration of activated eosinophils and mast cells. These activated cells, or activation of other cells, results in the release of allergen-provoked autacoids (such as histamine, prostaglandins and leukotrienes) and cytokines.

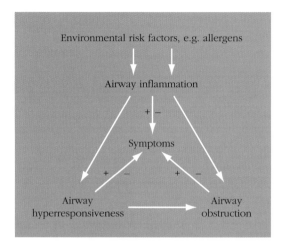

Figure 3.3 *Schematic representation of the interaction between airway inflammation, obstruction and hyperresponsiveness and asthma symptoms.*

Process of allergen sensitization

The mechanisms of airway inflammation involve a cascade of events including:

■ the process of sensitization to environmental allergen

■ IgE and T cell-driven release of inflammatory mediators, and

■ the recruitment of inflammatory cells from the circulation by increased expression (upregulation) of endothelial adhesion molecules (Figure 3.4).

Both of the functional divisions of the immune system, namely the B lymphocyte antibody-mediated and T lymphocyte cell-mediated immunity have important roles in airway inflammation of asthma. B lymphocytes produce specific antibodies (IgE) whilst T lymphocytes in addition to regulating B lymphocyte function, have proinflammatory actions through cytotoxic mechanisms and release of cytokines.

The real advances in asthma research have come in the last five to seven years, in the recognition of soluble markers called cytokines or interleukins which drive the inflammatory reaction and communicate the information between cells. In allergic asthma, this is initiated when allergen is identified by dendritic cells — antigen-presenting cells present in the bronchial epithelium — which present the allergen to

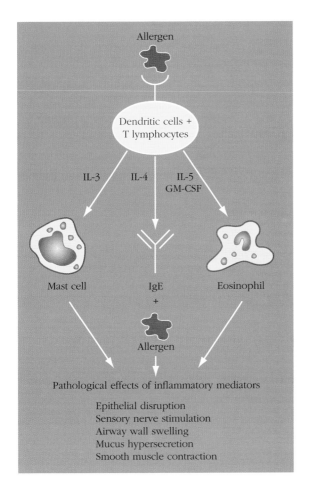

Figure 3.4 *The role of allergen, inflammatory, T lymphocytes and inflammatory mediators in asthma.*

the T lymphocyte in the airway. The T lymphocyte then starts to undergo differentiation and division in the local lymphoid tissue, then returns to the airway and presents the allergen to the B cell, which in the presence of certain of these soluble proteins, the interleukins, specifically interleukin 4[33] and 13[34], and helped by interleukin 6, inform the B cell to stop making immunoglobulin G and M and change it so that it synthesizes immunoglobulin E, the allergic antibody.

43

This is the process of sensitization. The next step is the linkage of this IgE onto the surface of the mediator-secreting cells by binding to receptors both of high (FcεR1) and of low (FcεR11) affinity on the surface of mast cells, basophils[35] and eosinophils. It is the cross-linking of this IgE on the surface of these cells that leads to the secretion of mediators. Not only are the autacoid mediators[36] released, causing the acute symptoms of asthma, but it is now recognized that these cells can generate newly formed interleukins that can support the B cell in the making of IgE and in addition can start recruiting eosinophils from the microvascular network. This we believe is what happens in the milder end of the asthma spectrum.

In more severe disease, what appears to happen is that the T cell starts to amplify this response which in itself generates large amounts of cytokine, the interleukins that drive the eosinophil response. The T cell then takes primacy over the mast cell.

In addition to their primary role in allergen presentation, dendritic cells may also have a role in maintaining the immune response once an individual is sensitized to allergen. Dendritic cells line the bronchi both in the epithelium and in the submucosa and are identified by the presence of a specific cell surface marker CD1a[+]. Recent evidence has shown that both high and low affinity receptors for IgE are present on the surface of dendritic cells[37] and these cells are increased in the bronchial epithelium of asthmatics, suggesting an IgE interaction in propagating the immune response.

Antigen presentation takes place in the bronchial lymphoid tissue and involves an interaction between dendritic cells and T lymphocytes resulting in differentiation along the Th2 pathway[38–41]. When activated by antigen, the Th2 cells result in direct synthesis of cytokines — IL-3, IL-4, IL-5, IL-9, IL-13 and GM-CSF (granulocyte macrophage-colony stimulating factor) — that directly results in leukocyte recruitment. In contrast, the Th1 cells differentiate in the presence of a different range of antigens associated with the delayed type IV hypersensitivity characteristic of diseases such as tuberculosis and sarcoidosis. Th1 cells generate predominantly interferon-γ (IFN-γ), IL-2, TNF-β and GM-CSF, which are protective.

The chain of events resulting in an inflammatory response of mast cell activation and eosinophil recruitment as a response to allergen sensitization is depicted in Figure 3.5.

Cellular biology of allergic airway inflammation

Following sensitization, the lower respiratory tract responds to inhaled allergen in a specific manner that results in airway obstruction and hyperresponsiveness. As described earlier, the EAR is a mast cell-dependent response resulting from IgE-dependent secretion of constrictor mediators: histamine, PGD2 and the sulphodipeptide leukotrienes LTC4 and LTD4. The late asthmatic reaction (LAR) ensues 2–6 hours after an antigen challenge and can persist for up to 24 hours. Until recently, it has been difficult to provide a cellular basis for the LAR, but in both animal models and more recently in human asthma, the LAR has been shown to occur in association with an influx of neutrophils and eosinophils into the airways. Bronchial biopsy specimens taken 4–6 hours after allergen challenge demonstrate:

- a significant increase in neutrophils, eosinophils and T lymphocytes within the submucosa and epithelium
- migration of mast cells towards the airway surface[42,43].

Perhaps of more importance are the mechanisms by which the leukocytes move into the airway and become activated. In addition to the pathological changes above, microscopic examination confirms that the leukocytes are seen to adhere to and migrate through the microvasculature. How do these eosinophil leukocytes, which we see in such large numbers in the lung, get into the lung? There have been some major advances in recent times. We know that in asthma, eosinophils are recruited from the blood vessels, the microvasculature of the airway. What appears to happen is that a group of molecules called adhesion molecules are upregulated on the luminal side of the microvascular bed, and these adhesion molecules grasp the leukocytes as they go by, and trap them in the presence of certain mediators[44,45]. This results in the generation of an array of molecules in sequence, that selectively recruit the eosinophil. We recognize now that the mast cell and the T lymphocyte secrete the soluble proteins that

45

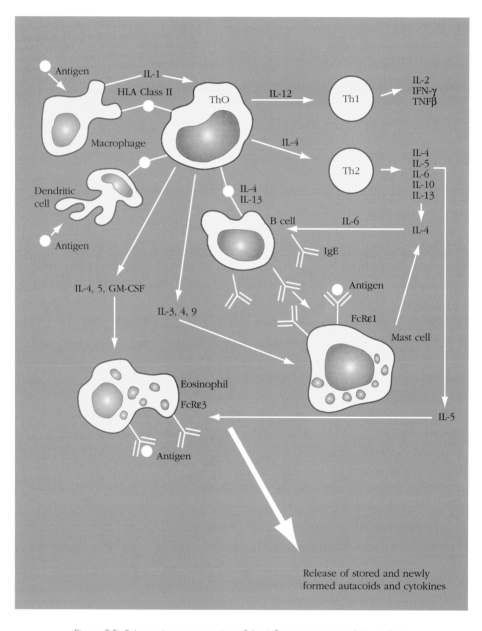

Figure 3.5 *Schematic representation of the inflammatory cascade in asthma.*

upregulate adhesion molecules and again it turns out that they are these interleukins or cytokines. What appears to happen is that the adhesion molecules [P-, L- and E-selectin, ICAM-1 (intercellular adhesion molecule-1) and VCAM 1 (vascular adhesion molecule-1)] are upregulated, the eosinophil is trapped against the endothelial cell with two or more of these molecules helping the eosinophil through the microvascular junctions and then, in the presence of a variety of these cytokines, the eosinophil migrates through the airway towards the airway surface. This is a process referred to as chemotaxis. Mediators are released on the way and this leads to disordered airway function and the symptoms of asthma.

The upregulation of the endothelial adhesion molecules is under the control of specific cytokines. E-selectin expression is upregulated by IL-1, TNF-α and IFN-γ. The same cytokines are also responsible for the upregulation of ICAM-1 whilst the optimal expression of VCAM-1 requires IL-4. The capacity of IL-4 to upregulate VCAM-1 expression on endothelial cells provides an important link with the early events following allergen challenge. Initially it was thought that T lymphocytes and monocytes were the prime source of the cytokines. Given that these cells require up to 6 hours to generate cytokines (*de novo*) prior to secretion[44], this would not explain the expression of E-selectin and ICAM-1 with the associated leukocyte influx that is already well established 6 hours after allergen challenge. Evidence from Southampton has shown that in biopsy specimens taken from subjects with asthma, IL-4, IL-5, IL-6 and TNF-α can be localized to mast cells[46]. Further support comes from the evidence that cross-linkage of mast cell-bound IgE releases both IL-4 and TNF-α in vast quantities that surpass the necessity to synthesize new protein and could account for the early upregulation of adhesion molecules. Thus, allergen-induced release of preformed TNF-α from mast cells could explain the observed upregulation of E-selectin and ICAM-1 during the LAR, with IL-5 augmenting eosinophil chemotaxis and IL-4 promoting eosinophil and T lymphocyte recruitment through its capacity to upregulate VCAM-1. These observations indicate a role for mast cells as early instigators of allergen-induced inflammation and, because Th2 cells also depend on IL-4 for their survival and proliferation, indicate a further role for mast cells in augmenting and prolonging T lymphocyte-dependent inflammation. When it is recognized that every mast cell will respond to allergen by releasing mediators, whereas only up to 1 in 2000 T lymphocytes are allergen specific[47], the role of the mast cell in orchestrating the allergic inflammatory response assumes more importance.

Non-allergic airway inflammation

It is now recognized that patients with asthma have persistent airway inflammation even in the absence of allergens, implying that factors other than mast cells and T lymphocytes are important in maintaining airway inflammation. Attention has focused on resident matrix (or constitutive) cells that are capable of contributing to the cytokine milieu that is not necessarily antigen-dependent. The epithelium is a source of IL-6, IL-8, IL-18, GM-CSF and TNF-α[48,49], whilst the endothelium can generate IL-5, IL-8 and GM-CSF. Fibroblasts are also an important source of the mast cell growth factor, *ckit*-ligand (stem cell or Steel factor), IL-8 and GM-CSF[50]. Together, these cytokines provide a non-allergic mechanism for initiating and maintaining the inflammatory response. Such mechanisms may be important in the chronic persistent form of asthma, and even in forms not associated with an initial allergic stimulus such as 'intrinsic' asthma. In 'extrinsic' or allergic asthma, withdrawal of environmental agents often produces only a partial remission, and it remains possible, therefore, that the chronicity of asthma is dependent upon inflammatory processes that are yet unrecognized and escape the control of the mucosal immune system.

In the past it has been believed that neurogenic inflammation, primarily through increased activity of the parasympathetic autonomic nervous system, could be important in the pathogenesis of asthma. In addition to the cholinergic and adrenergic pathways, a system of 'nonadrenergic–noncholinergic' (NANC) innervation has been described in human airways, with potent neuropeptides as neurotransmitters. Of these, substance P, calcitonin gene-related peptide (CGRP), vasoactive intestinal peptide (VIP) and neurokinins A and B (NKA and NKB) are the best characterized[51,52]. In addition to causing a vagally mediated bronchoconstriction, irritant stimuli, such as acid aerosols, dust and cold air, stimulate the airway sensory nerves via non-myelinated C-fibre endings to release neuropeptides, that contribute to some of the characteristic pathological effects of asthma, such as smooth muscle contraction, mucus hypersecretion and, perhaps most importantly, inflammatory cell activation. It is the latter effect that has revived interest in possible abnormalities of the neural control of airways in the 'non-allergic' pathogenesis of asthma. Furthermore, VIP is thought to act as a cotransmitter with acetylcholine in efferent cholinergic nerves in the airway, with a presumed role in limiting cholinergic bronchoconstriction. Peptidases released from eosinophils, mast cells and neutrophils have the capacity to degrade VIP with the result of exaggerating reflex cholinergic bronchoconstriction. Nitric oxide (NO), the presumed neurotransmitter of NANC inhibitory nerves, has also recently received attention[53,54], although abnormalities in the metabolism of NO and its role in the pathophysiology of asthma remains to be established. Based on current knowledge, abnormalities in the neural control of the airways are important, although they are not recognized as a major cause of the airway hyperresponsiveness and obstruction seen in allergic and non-allergic asthma.

Role of current treatment in airway inflammation

A better understanding of the mechanisms of allergen-provoked early and late phase responses has helped to explain how various drugs operate in asthma. By inhibiting the release of pre-formed and newly generated autacoids from activated mast cells, both nedocromil sodium and sodium cromoglycate inhibit the early and late phase responses and acquired bronchial hyperresponsiveness. Oral and topical corticosteroids reduce the late response probably by inhibiting the cytokine-mediated upregulation of adhesion molecules on microvasculature, in addition to their effect in reducing cytokine secretion from mast cells and T lymphocytes. The effect of beta-2 agonists largely relates to their specific influence on mast cells and

49

their capacity to antagonize the constrictor properties of mast cell and eosinophil-derived mediators, such as histamine.

Role of future treatment in airway inflammation

Activated neutrophils and eosinophils once recruited into the airways, secrete an array of inflammatory mediators and cytokines. These include the toxic granule components of the eosinophil, e.g. major basic protein (MBP) and eosinophil cationic protein (ECP) and a range of lipid products including leukotrienes and platelet-activating factor (PAF). Availability of potent and selective leukotriene antagonists has been useful as medication[55,56] and in dissecting the contribution of the mediators in the EAR and LAR. Prior administration of LTD4 antagonists before allergen challenge has conferred a marked inhibitory effect, not only on the EAR and LAR, but also on the acquired increase in BHR. Some of these drugs are available in some countries and their therapeutic potential will be identified in due course. Early research supports management of aspirin-induced asthma with leukotriene-receptor antagonists or inhibitors of leukotriene generation. Although PAF was once regarded as a prime mediator of the LAR and BHR, trials with orally active PAF antagonists have been less encouraging with no inhibitory effects demonstrated either on the EAR or LAR[57]. Potent antagonists of other mast cell-derived mediators are also currently under investigation, namely tryptase, the predominant neutral protease secreted by the mast cell.

Based on the current evidence of airway inflammation in asthma, the national and international guidelines that emphasize the early treatment of asthma with anti-inflammatory therapy clearly have an important role. Recognizing the importance of airway inflammation has profound implications in terms of disease management and prevention. The observation that inflammation is present in the airways of asthmatics with intermittent or mild symptoms raises the question as to whether the disease should be treated with anti-inflammatory agents irrespective of clinical severity. Whether early intervention can affect the progression of intermittent asthma to the chronic condition will be determined by long-term studies of the effects of treatment including side effects. Furthermore, the view that severe chronic asthma is tightly linked to airway dysfunction owing to inflammation has recently been challenged: a bronchial biopsy and lavage study of patients on high-dose inhaled corticosteroids has shown that, when compared to mild asthmatics, the steroid-treated group had fewer activated T lymphocytes and eosinophils, yet had marked airway hyperresponsiveness and symptoms[58]. In another biopsy study in children and young atopic adults taking large doses of oral corticosteroids (up to 60 mg), patients showed marked T lymphocyte activation and eosinophil infiltration, and increased mRNA expression of IL-5 and IL-13[59]. These observations suggest that, in severe asthma, factors other than mucosal inflammation may be contributing to airway dysfunction, and that these appear to escape the anti-inflammatory effects of corticosteroids.

It is clear that future treatment strategies should be based on recognizing and inhibiting the underlying airway inflammation rather than treating the symptoms alone. This can be enhanced by increasing our understanding of the mechanisms underlying acute and chronic inflammation; this may explain why the inflammatory response is not attenuated after anti-inflammatory therapy in all patients with asthma.

References

1 Salter H. *On asthma: its pathology and treatment* (2nd edn). London: Churchill, 1868.

2 Osler W. *The principles and practice of medicine.* New York: Appleton, 1892.

3 Holgate ST. Asthma: past, present and future. The 1992 Cournand Lecture. *Eur Resp J* 1993; **6**: 1507–20.

4 Djukanovic R, Roche WR, Wilson JW *et al.* Mucosal inflammation in asthma. *Am Rev Resp Dis* 1990; **142**: 434–57.

5 Global Initiative for Asthma. *Global strategy for asthma management and prevention. NHLBI/WHO Workshop.* National Heart, Lung and Blood Institute, Publication No. 95-3659, January 1995.

6 Woolcock AJ, Salome CM, Yan K. The shape of the dose–response to histamine in asthmatic and normal subjects. *Am Rev Resp Dis* 1984; **130**: 71–5.

7 Hargreave FE, Pizzichini MM, Pizzichini E. Airway hyperresponsiveness as a diagnostic feature of asthma. In: Johansson SGO, ed. *Progress in allergy and clinical immunology.* Vol. 3. Stockholm: Hogrefe and Huber Publishers, 1995.

8 Pattemore PK, Holgate ST. Bronchial hyperresponsiveness and its relationship to asthma in childhood. *Clin Exp Allergy* 1993; **23**: 886–900.

9 Salome CM, Peat JK, Britton WJ, Woolcock AJ. Bronchial hyperresponsiveness in two populations of Australian schoolchildren. *Clin Allergy* 1987; **17**: 271–81.

10 Sears MR, Jones DT, Holdaway MD *et al.* Prevalence of bronchial hyper-reactivity to inhaled methacholine in New Zealand children. *Thorax* 1986; **41**: 283–89.

11 Pattemore PK, Asher MI, Harrison AC, Rea HH, Stewart AW. The interrelationship among bronchial hyperresponsiveness, the diagnosis of asthma, and asthma symptoms. *Am Rev Resp Dis* 1990; **142**: 549–54.

12 Pin I, Radford S, Kolendowicz R *et al.* Airway inflammation in symptomatic and asymptomatic children with methacholine hyperresponsiveness. *Eur Resp J* 1993; **6**: 1249–56.

13 Brand PLP, Rijekan B, Shouten JP, Koeter GH, Weiss ST, Postma DS. Perception of airway obstruction in a random population sample. Relationship to airway hyperresponsiveness in the absence of respiratory symptoms. *Am Rev Resp Dis* 1992; **146**: 396–401.

14 Hargreave FE, Ramsdale EH, Pugsley SO. Occupational asthma without bronchial hyperresponsiveness. *Am Rev Resp Dis* 1984; **130**: 513–15.

15 Ryan G, Latimer KM, Dolovich J, Hargreave F. Bronchial responsiveness to histamine: relationship to diurnal variation of peak flow rate, improvement after bronchodilator, and airway calibre. *Thorax* 1982; **37**: 423–9.

16 Holgate ST. Mediator and cytokine mechanisms in asthma [Altounyan address]. *Thorax* 1993; **48**: 103–9.

17 Triggiani M, Cirillo R, Lichtenstein LM, Marone G. Inhibition of histamine and prostaglandin D2 release from human lung mast cells by ciclosporin A. *Int Arch Allergy Appl Immunol* 1989; **88**: 253–5.

18 Friedman BS, Bel EH, Buntinx A *et al.* Oral leukotriene inhibitor (MK-886) blocks allergen-induced airway responses. *Am Rev Resp Dis* 1993; **147**: 839–44.

19 Al Jarad N, Hui KP, Barnes N. Effects of a thromboxane receptor antagonist on prostaglandin D2 and histamine induced bronchoconstriction in man. *Br J Clin Pharmacol* 1994; **37**: 97–100.

20 Hui KP, Taylor IK, Taylor GW *et al.* Effect of a 5-lipoxygenase inhibitor on leukotriene generation and airway responses after allergen challenge in asthmatic patients. *Thorax* 1991; **46**: 184–189.

21 Curzen N, Rafferty P, Holgate ST. Effects of a cyclo-oxygenase inhibitor, flurbiprofen, and an H1 histamine receptor antagonist, terfenadine, alone and in combination on allergen induced immediate bronchoconstriction in man. *Thorax* 1987; **42**: 946–52.

22 Beasley CRW, Robinson C, Featherstone RL *et al.* 9α,11β-Prostaglandin F2, a novel metabolite of prostaglandin D2, is a potent contractile agonist of human and guinea pig airways. *J Clin Invest* 1987; **79**: 978–83.

23 Roche WR, Beasley R, Williams JH, Holgate ST. Subepithelial fibrosis in the bronchi of asthmatics. *Lancet* 1989; **i**: 520–4.

24 Brewster CEP, Howarth PH, Djukanovic R, Wilson J, Holgate ST, Roche WR. Myofibroblasts and subepithelial fibrosis in bronchial asthma. *Am J Resp Cell Mol Biol* 1990; **3**: 507–11.

25 James AL, Par PD, Hogg JC. The mechanics of airway narrowing in asthma. *Am Rev Resp Dis* 1989; **139**: 242–6.

26 Gleich GJ, Flavahan NA, Fujisawa T, Vanhoutte PM. The eosinophil as a mediator of damage to respiratory epithelium: a model for bronchial hyperreactivity. *J Allergy Clin Immunol* 1988; **81**: 776–81.

27 Montefort S, Baker J, Roche WR, Holgate ST. The distribution of adhesive mechanisms in the normal bronchial epithelium. *Eur Resp J* 1993; **6**: 1257–63.

28 Sillaber C, Strobl H, Bevec D *et al.* IL-4 regulates *c-kit* proto-oncogene product expression in human mast and myeloid progenitor cells. *J Immunol* 1991; **147**: 4224–8.

29 Vilcek J, Palombella VJ, Henrikson-DeStefano D *et al.* Fibroblast growth enhancing activity of tumor necrosis factor and its relationship to other polypeptide growth factors. *J Exp Med* 1986; **163**: 632–43.

30 Aubert JD, Dalal BI, Bai TR, Roberts CR, Hayashi S, Hogg JC. Transforming growth factor beta 1 gene expression in human airways. *Thorax* 1994; **49**: 225–32.

31 Moreno RH, Hogg JC, Par PD. Mechanics of airway narrowing. *Am Rev Resp Dis* 1986; **133**: 1171–80.

32 Wiggs BR, Bosken C, Par PD, James A, Hogg JC. A model of airway narrowing in asthma and in chronic obstructive pulmonary disease. *Am Rev Resp Dis* 1992; **145**: 1251–8.

33 Del Prete G, Maggi E, Parronchi P *et al.* IL-4 is an essential factor for the IgE synthesis induced in vitro by human T cell clones and their supernatants. *J Immunol* 1988; **140**: 4193–8.

34 McKenzie ANJ, Culpepper JA, de Waal Malefyt R *et al.* Interleukin 13, a T-cell-derived cytokine that regulates human monocyte and B-cell function. *Proc Nat Acad Sci USA* 1993; **90**: 3735–9.

35 Gauchat J-F, Henchoz S, Mazzel G *et al.* Induction of human IgE synthesis in B cells by mast cells and basophils. *Nature* 1993; **365**: 340–3.

36 Kay AB. Asthma and inflammation. *J Allergy Clin Immunol* 1991; **87**: 893–910.

37 Tunon de Lara JM, Bradding P, Redington AE, Church MK, Holgate ST. Dendritic cells (DCs) in asthmatic airways express the high affinity receptor for IgE. *Am J Resp Critical Care Med* 1994; **149**: A958 (Abs.).

38 Del Prete GF, De Carli M, D'Elios MM *et al.* Allergen exposure induces the activation of allergen-specific Th2 cells in the airway mucosa of patients with allergic respiratory disorders. *Eur J Immunol* 1993; **23**: 1445–9.

39 Mosmann TR, Coffman RL. TH1 and TH2 cells: different patterns of lymphokine secretion lead to different functional properties. *A Rev Immunol* 1989; **7**: 145–73.

40 Robinson DS, Hamid Q, Ying S *et al.* Predominant TH2-like bronchoalveolar T-lymphocyte population in atopic asthma. *New Engl J Med* 1992; **326**: 298–304.

41 Burd PR, Rogers HW, Gordon JR *et al.* Interleukin 3-dependent and -independent mast cells stimulated with IgE and antigen express multiple cytokines. *J Exp Med* 1989; **170**: 245–7.

42 Montefort S, Gratziou C, Goulding D *et al.* Bronchial biopsy evidence for leukocyte infiltration and upregulation of leukocyte-endothelial cell adhesion molecules 6 hours after local allergen challenge of sensitized asthmatic airways. *J Clin Invest* 1994; **93**: 1411–21.

43 Gratziou C, Carroll M, Walls A, Howarth PH, Holgate ST. Early changes in T lymphocytes recovered by bronchoalveolar lavage after local allergen challenge of asthmatic airways. *Am Rev Resp Dis* 1992; **145**: 1259–64.

44 Springer TA. Adhesion receptors of the immune system. *Nature* 1990; **346**: 425–34.

45 Montefort S, Holgate ST, Howarth PH. Leucocyte-endothelial adhesion molecules and their role in bronchial asthma and allergic rhinitis. *Eur Resp J* 1993; **6**: 1044–54.

46 Bradding P, Feather IH, Howarth PH *et al.* Interleukin 4 is localized to and released by human mast cells. *J Exp Med* 1992; **176**: 1381–6.

47 Corrigan CJ, Baiqing L, Durham SR, Kay AB. Allergen-specific T lymphocytes selectively accumulate in the airways of atopic non-asthmatics. *Am J Resp Critical Care Med* 1994; **149**: A951 (Abs.).

48 Bellini A, Yoshimura H, Vittori E, Marini M, Mattoli S. Bronchial epithelial cells of patients with asthma release chemoattractant factors for T lymphocytes. *J Allergy Clin Immunol* 1993; **92**: 412–24.

49 Devalia JL, Campbell AM, Sapsford RJ *et al.* Effect of nitrogen dioxide on synthesis of inflammatory cytokines expressed by human bronchial epithelial cells in vitro. *Am J Resp Cell Mol Biol* 1993; **9**: 271–8.

50 Vancheri C, Gauldie J, Bienenstock J *et al.* Human lung fibroblast-derived granulocyte macrophage colony stimulating factor (GM-CSF) mediates eosinophil survival in vitro. *Am J Resp Cell Mol Biol* 1989; **1**: 289–95.

51 Barnes PJ, Baraniuk JN, Belvisi MG. Neuropeptides in the respiratory tract Part I. *Am Rev Resp Dis* 1991; **144**: 1187–98.

52 Barnes PJ, Baraniuk JN, Belvisi MG. Neuropeptides in the respiratory tract Part II. *Am Rev Resp Dis* 1991; **144**: 1391–9.

53 Hamid Q, Springall DR, Riveros-Moreno V *et al.* Induction of nitric oxide synthase in asthma. *Lancet* 1993; **342**: 1510–13.

54 Robbins RA, Barnes PJ, Springall DR *et al.* Expression of inducible nitric oxide synthase in human lung epithelial cells. *Biochem Biophys Res Commun* 1994; **203**: 209–18.

55 Cloud ML, Enas GC, Kemp J *et al.* A specific LTD4/LTE4 antagonist improves pulmonary function in patients with mild, chronic asthma. *Am Rev Resp Dis* 1989; **140**: 1336–9.

56 Smith LJ, Geller S, Ebright L, Glass M, Thyrum PT. Inhibition of leukotriene D4-induced bronchoconstriction in normal subjects by the oral LTD4 receptor antagonist ICI 204,219. *Am Rev Resp Dis* 1990; **141**: 988–92.

57 Kuitert LM, Hui KP, Uthayarkumaar S *et al.* Effect of the platelet-activating factor antagonist UK-74,505 on the early and late response to allergen. *Am Rev Resp Dis* 1993; **147**: 82–6.

58 Redington AE, Britten KM, Walls AF *et al.* Airway inflammatory changes in chronic corticosteroid treated symptomatic asthma. *J Allergy Clin Immunol* 1995 (in press).

59 Vrugt B, Wilson S, Underwood JM *et al.* Increased expression of interleukin-2 receptor in peripheral blood and bronchial biopsies from severe asthmatics. *Eur Resp J* 1994; **7**: 239s.

Chapter 4

Diagnosis

Making the diagnosis and using the term 'asthma' are fundamental to the effective management of asthma. The diagnostic process begins with awareness of the symptom complexes associated with asthma, followed by confirmation using lung function tests, usually peak expiratory flow (PEF), and a trial of therapy.

Community-based studies have consistently shown that asthma is underdiagnosed in children[1-7] and adults[8,9]. It is vital to make the diagnosis because undiagnosed asthmatic children are inappropriately treated[7,10]. Early diagnosis is important because there is some evidence[11,12] that earlier treatment of asthma with anti-inflammatory medication may be of benefit. Furthermore, it has recently been suggested that permanent lung damage may result from undertreated asthma[13]; this adds further justification to the rationale for earlier treatment with anti-inflammatory medication. Therefore, early diagnosis is a major goal for asthma care in the community as this may substantially reduce morbidity. Avoidable morbidity in childhood asthma is due to three main factors (see box).

Without using the term 'asthma', it is not possible to provide our patients with rational treatment, appropriate educational advice and self-management plans. Diagnosis of asthma is fairly straightforward in older children and younger adults; however, there are major difficulties in diagnosing children under 5 years of age and elderly patients. There is currently much debate regarding the taxonomy of young children with intermittent wheezing illness that is often due to

Causes of avoidable morbidity in childhood asthma

Diagnosis
- incorrect
- delayed

Treatment
- inappropriate choice of drug
- inappropriate dose or frequency
- inappropriate choice of inhaler

Education
- not given
- not understood
- not followed (non-compliance)

virus infections. Which wheezy infants later go on to develop asthma and how many will 'outgrow it' are other current unanswered questions. The prognosis is related to the severity and frequency of wheezing episodes[14]. In infants (children under 1 year old) it was agreed in the latest version of the BTS guidelines[15] that it is acceptable to use the terms 'wheezing illness' or 'infantile asthma' in order to avoid disagreement in trying to define asthma in this age group. The younger the wheezy child the more important it is to consider referral to a paediatrician in order to exclude other possible diagnoses. Diagnostic difficulties also arise in elderly patients where problems occur in differentiating asthma from chronic obstructive pulmonary disease, which often coexists.

In this chapter we discuss the problems associated with diagnosing asthma, including delayed and underdiagnosis, unusual presentations, specialist investigations and differential diagnoses. Finally we describe some practical ways in which readers may enhance their diagnostic skills in asthma, resulting in earlier diagnosis.

The diagnosis of asthma

The typically asthmatic patient presents repeatedly with respiratory symptoms. It is the recurrent nature of these presentations that should alert the clinician. In most of these cases, making the diagnosis depends entirely on obtaining a detailed history of symptoms from the patients and in the case of children from their parents, followed by objective confirmation with lung function tests such as peak expiratory flow (PEF) and spirometry measurements.

Delayed diagnosis

There is often a long delay between the onset of respiratory symptoms and the diagnosis of asthma in children[4,17,18]. However, this delay does seem to be reducing in the UK[19,20]. The delay in diagnosis could possibly be explained by the nature of general practice in the National Health Service:

■ long delays in obtaining past medical records
■ poor continuity of care which results from mobility of patients
■ doctors working in larger group practices where patients consult different doctors each time they attend, and
■ a general reluctance by doctors and patients to use the term 'asthma'[21].

A lack of awareness of the presenting symptoms of asthma (see box) might also explain the delay in diagnosis in primary care[22,23]. Many children attend their general practitioner with recurrent episodes of 'cough', 'bronchitis' or 'chest infections' before the diagnosis of asthma is considered[1,4,6,24].

Symptoms

Recurrent wheeze, cough, breathlessness and chest tightness are the commonest symptoms suggestive of asthma in children and adults. Initial presentation with one or more of these symptoms may occur at any age (termed 'late-onset asthma' if in adulthood). There are many other causes of these symptoms in childhood (Table 4.1).

Presenting symptoms of asthma in general practice

Well-known

■ cough
   'still coughing'
   'coughing for months'
   'no better despite antibiotics'
   'worse when laughing'
   'induced by exercise'
■ wheeze
■ shortness of breath
■ chest tightness

Less well-known

■ difficulty in sleeping
■ spoilt holiday
■ chest pain
■ vomiting
■ itching (children, usually preceding attacks, usually upper body)

In trying to establish a diagnosis in children, health professionals often depend on the parents' description of symptoms. However, some parents are unclear what wheeze sounds like, and mistake rattley breathing from upper airway secretions or even stridor for wheeze. Recurrent cough, especially at night or with exercise, is reported more commonly than wheeze, especially in preschool asthmatic children. In adults, cardiac or respiratory problems such as cardiac failure, recurrent pulmonary emboli may present with recurrent respiratory symptoms that mimic asthma (Table 4.1)

The diagnosis of asthma is supported by a history that the symptoms are precipitated by particular trigger factors (see box).

Minor viral upper respiratory tract infections in the younger child and exercise in the older child are the most common and easily

Table 4.1 Causes of recurrent respiratory symptoms

Causes	Frequency
In young children	
Asthma	Very common
Idiopathic	Very common
Following viral bronchiolitis	Common
Maternal smoking (ante- +/- postnatal)	Common
Prematurity +/- neonatal lung disease	Uncommon
Recurrent aspiration of feeds	Uncommon
Congenital lung/heart defects	Uncommon
Cystic fibrosis	Uncommon
Inhaled foreign body	Uncommon
Immunodeficiency	Very uncommon
In adults	
Asthma	Very common
Cardiac failure	Uncommon
Recurrent pulmonary emboli	Common
Following upper and lower respiratory viral infections	Common

---

Trigger factors for asthma

- Viral infections
- Exercise
- Allergen exposure
- Cigarette smoke
- Emotional upset
- Chemical irritants
- Cold air
- Occupational exposure

---

recognized triggers in childhood. Viral infections, emotional upset or excitement, sudden changes in temperature or humidity, exposure to common allergens such as cats, dogs or grass pollens, and the inhalation of chemical irritants such as cigarette smoke or domestic aerosols, are important triggers for older children and adults.

Elderly patients pose particular diagnostic (and therapeutic) problems in asthma because there are often other concomitant diseases present. Asthma in the elderly is underdiagnosed[25] and therefore undertreated. In some elderly patients the respiratory symptoms are non-specific, physical examination may be unhelpful and the ability to do PEF readings impaired. In these circumstances spirometry may be more helpful, or failing this, the response to a trial of therapy.

The statement 'all that wheezes is asthma until proved otherwise' is a useful guide in childhood but it is important to be aware that other conditions, such as cystic fibrosis, bronchiolitis and inhaled foreign bodies, may present as wheeze and need to be clearly identified. There is a group of children under the age of 2 who regularly wheeze, do not respond well to treatment but who thrive normally and grow out of their symptoms without developing asthma. In the older age groups symptoms in patients with chronic obstructive airways disease, mitral valve disease and bronchiectasis (see Chapter 7) may be confused with asthma. It is important the correct diagnosis is reached by appropriate investigation to ensure proper management.

More difficult to manage are patients with definite asthma, often of mild degree, who also have significant psychological problems and who present with frequent acute hyperventilation/panic attacks. Many of these patients show peak flows which swing wildly, often associated with mood changes, there being no logical pattern. They respond poorly to corticosteroids. This pattern may start in adolescence and unless handled firmly may lead to a patient being kept on large doses of oral steroids with the potential for side effects in the long term.

Atopic disease as an indicator of asthma in childhood

A third of children with asthma have also had eczema. Over 50% will have the symptoms of allergic rhinitis, with recurrent or persistent obstruction of the nostrils, sniffing, sneezing and nasal discharge. There may be accompanying redness and swelling of the eyes (allergic conjunctivitis). These symptoms may occur only in the summer when the grass pollen count is high ('hay-fever') or throughout the year (perennial rhinitis). Children with asthma are three to four times more likely to have a parent or sibling with atopic disease than non-asthmatic children: if one parent has atopic disease, the child has a 50% risk of developing an atopic disorder, and if both parents are atopic, then the risk to the child is 70%. However, the absence of a personal or family history of atopy does not preclude the diagnosis of asthma.

The associations between asthma and recurrent croup or urticaria are less well recognized (see box). Recurrent (or spasmodic) croup is a syndrome of inspiratory stridor, a barking cough and difficulty in breathing. Characteristically, there is acute onset of these symptoms at night. Recurrent croup is more common in children with a personal or family history of atopic disease.

Examination

In many patients with asthma, the physical examination is normal when they are seen in the surgery or outpatient clinic. It is vital to appreciate that the absence of abnormal signs does not preclude the diagnosis of asthma. In some patients, there will be hyperinflation, with an increased anteroposterior diameter of the chest, or expiratory wheeze. The presence of a chest deformity, such as Harrison's sulci or pectus carinatum, usually indicates long-standing and marked airways obstruction. Wheeze or crackles that are consistently present in only one area of the lung suggest focal lung disease such as infection, an inhaled foreign body, bronchiectasis, or a tumour in older patients. Finger clubbing is not a feature of

---

Atopic diseases in childhood

- Asthma
- Eczema
- Allergic rhinitis
- Allergic conjunctivitis
- Recurrent croup
- Urticaria

asthma: its presence indicates another diagnosis. The skin should be examined for eczema, and the nasal mucosa for the features of allergic rhinitis.

In children height and weight should be measured accurately and plotted on the appropriate percentile chart. Except in severe uncontrolled asthma, growth is normal; abnormal growth suggests there may be another cause of symptoms, such as cystic fibrosis or immunodeficiency.

Unusual presentations and difficult diagnosis of asthma

Some asthmatic patients of all ages never (or seldom) wheeze: they suffer from recurrent coughing. This condition is termed 'cough variant asthma'. It is characterized by a persistent, non-productive cough with minimal or no wheezing and dyspnoea, but normal lung function tests, and may often resolve with anti-asthma treatment[26,27]. A review of 15 clinically orientated research articles revealed a variable natural history of cough variant asthma. While a significant proportion of these patients eventually develop the classic signs and symptoms of asthma, many resolve without the need for further treatment[26,27]. Other unusual symptoms of asthma include recurrent vomiting[26,28] and itching[29,30]. The latter is fairly common in children, usually affects the upper part of the body and often precedes an exacerbation of asthma (prodromal itching).

Preschool children: Diagnosing asthma in preschool children can be difficult as there is no satisfactory definition that can be used in clinical practice. Because these children are too young to perform even the simplest lung function tests, there is no objective evidence of variable airflow obstruction. Another difficulty in this age group is that wheezing in young children is not necessarily due to asthma. One working definition of preschool asthma is: 'Any preschool child who has had at least three episodes of wheezing and has an atopic first degree relative is likely to have asthma.'

Occupational asthma: 'Occupational asthma is due wholly or partly to agents met with at work'[31]. The true prevalence of occupational asthma is unknown and the compensation figures obtainable from different government bodies underestimate the actual occurrence of this disease entity[31]. Occupational asthma may result primarily from exposure at work or may develop secondarily in previously diagnosed asthmatics. The main clue to the diagnosis is that symptoms are worse on workdays and improve when patients are off duty or on holiday. Serial PEF measurements, taken over several weeks, (every few hours, from waking to sleeping) often lead to the diagnosis of occupational asthma[32]. It is extremely important to make the diagnosis in these cases because the patient may improve (and others will be protected) if the causative agent is removed from the workplace. Unfortunately the asthma may not resolve completely even if the patient is withdrawn completely from exposure. Anyone who has developed occupational asthma may be eligible for compensation and it would be advisable to refer the patient either to an occupational physician or a respiratory physician with an interest in occupational medicine.

Elderly patients: In contrast to younger patients where measurement and calculation of variability using peak flow meters is acceptable, spirometry may be of greater help in diagnosing asthma in the elderly[33]. There is, however, no agreement on the best measures of variability and this is compounded by the availability of limited information on normal or predicted values of lung function measurements. Dow[33] suggests that the FEV_1/FVC ratio is the best criterion because, if the FVC and the FEV_1 are taken into account, patients who have mixed restrictive and obstructive lung disease will be correctly diagnosed. Those patients who have an FEV_1/FVC ratio below 60% have obstructive airways disease and should be offered a trial of anti-asthma therapy. Those with normal or near normal lung function should be further investigated by recording twice daily peak flow measurements (Figs 4.1, 4.2).

Figure 4.1 *Peak flow chart.*
(3M Pharmaceuticals, with permission.)

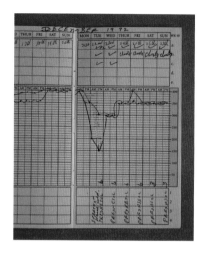

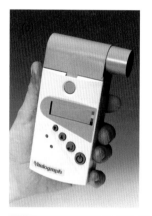

Figure 4.2 *Examples of spirometers*
(a, b) and a spirometry and flow volume
loop tracing (c).

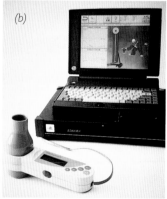

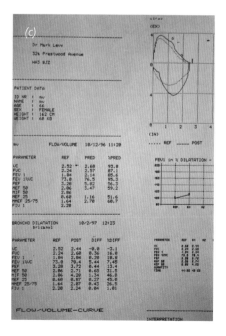

Variability >15–20% in PEF or FEV$_1$ is probably due to asthma. A significant proportion of adults over the age of 65 are unable to perform reliable spirometry or PEF and therefore the diagnosis of asthma may need to be made on the basis of symptoms (perhaps with appropriate quality of life measures[34–40]) and a trial of therapy. In determining a response to a trial of therapy, there are difficulties in interpreting variability based upon FEV$_1$ alone and therefore some specialists recommend using an absolute increase in FEV$_1$ of 200 ml[25]. It is important to note that demonstrating a response in elderly patients to bronchodilators alone is insufficient evidence upon which to base a decision to treat with inhaled steroids (Nissar *et al.*, 1990, quoted in Dow[25]). A trial of therapy with oral steroids in these patients is necessary to identify those patients who will benefit from long-term therapy with inhaled steroids. Patients with smoking-related airflow obstruction may not gain any additional benefit from the addition of inhaled steroids to bronchodilator treatment.

Differential diagnosis

Although 40% of children with asthma will have recurrent wheeze before the age of 2, many other disorders present with similar symptoms in this age group. Recurrent wheeze and cough are more common in preterm infants, in those with a history of bronchopulmonary dysplasia and, most frequently, in those following viral bronchiolitis. Children with gastro-oesophageal reflux, cystic fibrosis and congenital lung or cardiac anomalies can have similar symptoms. In many wheezy infants it is not possible to identify a definite cause, although it is probable that viral infections play an important role. The infants of mothers who smoke are twice as likely to have recurrent cough and wheeze as the children of non-smokers. These other causes should be carefully considered in the assessment of the young child with wheeze and, if there is any doubt, referral for appropriate assessment and investigations should be arranged.

In the elderly, the differentiation of chronic obstructive airways disease from asthma is difficult as the two may coexist. There is also a view that long-standing poorly controlled asthma may progress to 'irreversible' airways obstruction consequent upon airway wall remodelling. The FEV_1/FVC ratio is of help and a trial of therapy with oral or inhaled steroids is often necessary. Cardiac disease causing difficulty in breathing needs to be differentiated from asthma and a past medical or family history of heart disease may be helpful. Previous history of smoking or occupational exposure to substances injurious to the lungs may be of help in diagnosing other respiratory diseases.

Investigations

Initial investigations and confirmation of the diagnosis

In the older child with normal growth, and adults who have only respiratory or atopic symptoms, there is rarely any doubt that recurrent cough, wheeze and/or breathlessness are due to asthma. A trial of asthma therapy may be used to confirm the diagnosis. If the symptoms improve with bronchodilator therapy, or a trial of anti-inflammatory treatment, and if they reappear when this treatment is stopped, then asthma is the likely diagnosis.

Peak expiratory flow measurements and spirometry: The diagnosis of asthma can be confirmed by tests which demonstrate reversible airflow obstruction. This can often be demonstrated in the surgery or outpatient clinic, by measuring the peak expiratory flow (PEF) before, and 15 minutes after, inhalation of a beta-2 adrenergic-bronchodilator (such as salbutamol or terbutaline) (see box).

Inability to demonstrate reversible airflow obstruction does not exclude the diagnosis of asthma at this stage. Alternatively, a twice-daily record card of PEF (before and after treatment if appropriate), measured and recorded by the patient at home, often confirms the diagnosis. A change in readings of 15% from day to day, morning to evening or before and after bronchodilator treatment, would help to confirm the diagnosis of asthma (Figure 4.1). Most children over the age of 5 can perform peak flow measurements reliably.

Airflow variability can be demonstrated with the use of peak flow meters or spirometers. Peak flow meters range from cheap, hand-held

Reversibility test to diagnose variable airflow obstruction

1. Measure the patient's peak expiratory flow (PEF).
2. Administer two puffs of a beta-2 agonist bronchodilator (Ventolin, salbutamol, Bricanyl, terbutaline, preferably with a large volume spacer device).
3. Ask the patient to wait in the waiting room while the next patient may be seen.
4. After 15–20 minutes, measure the PEF again.
5. Calculate the variability by using the formula:

$$\frac{\text{Highest PEF} - \text{Lowest PEF}}{\text{Highest PEF}} \times 100$$

If the variability is >15% and the history suggests asthma, confirm the diagnosis!

portables (three of which are currently prescribable on the NHS Drug Tariff)[11], to more expensive electronic logging devices. Spirometers are available in a minority of general practice surgeries. Most asthmatic patients can be diagnosed and effectively managed using the cheaper meters. There are some problems related to the lack of adequate standardization of the meters in the UK. In practice this means that in order to achieve the most consistency in advising patients as well as self-help management, the patients should use their own meter to measure their PEF. Other countries have adopted a different approach, through the use of a different scale on the meters which renders the readings more accurate in terms of reference to those obtained by a pneumotachograph, which is the accepted gold standard.

Spirometry if available may be helpful in diagnosing asthma in a small proportion of patients whose PEF does not vary by more than 15%.

A variation over 15 to 20% is regarded as abnormal and, in combination with a suggestive history of asthma, confirms the diagnosis (see box). This is best done by asking the patient to keep a PEF diary for a few weeks, recording the best of three readings in the early morning, and ideally three in the late afternoon (or early evening if this is not possible). The degree of variability provides both a confirmation of the diagnosis as well as an indication of the severity of the patient's asthma: the higher the variability the more unstable the disease.

Further investigations

More detailed investigations are indicated only in a minority of older children and adults with severe or atypical asthma, as they add little to the management of the majority of cases. However these may be helpful in the differential diagnosis, recognition of unusual causes of asthma, management of acute attacks and in epidemiological and research studies. In over 90% of cases of childhood asthma, no investigations are necessary. If the diagnosis is in doubt, patients should be referred to a specialist respiratory physician or paediatrician for further investigation.

Use of peak expiratory flow readings in asthma

- For establishing the diagnosis
- For identifying causal factors:
    occupational triggers
    specific triggers, e.g. allergy
- To demonstrate the degree of reversibility
- In simple exercise testing
- For demonstrating response to treatment
- To determine optimal function
- As an indicator of failing control

Chest X-ray: A chest X-ray should be performed only if there is doubt about the diagnosis or if the symptoms are severe or persist after treatment. In the majority of cases of well controlled asthma, the chest X-ray is normal, but in severe chronic and acute asthma the films may demonstrate hyperinflated lung fields with low flat diaphragms and splaying of the ribs (Figure 4.3).

In children under 2 years of age, with persistent respiratory symptoms and respiratory distress, a chest X-ray is useful to exclude other causes of these symptoms. In the rare patients with asthma secondary to allergic bronchopulmonary aspergillosis, acute episodes may be associated with patchy shadowing or consolidation that may be at the same or different sites and resolve spontaneously or with oral steroids. In time this can lead to increased lung markings and fibrosis with the development of proximal bronchiectasis seen on CT scanning. In an acute asthma attack, a chest X-ray is not indicated unless there is clinical evidence of infection or deterioration in the patient's condition, when it may reveal collapse, consolidation,

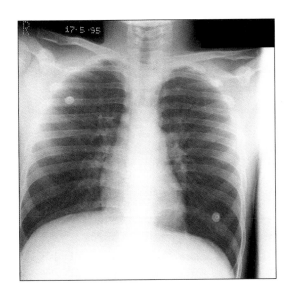

Figure 4.3 *Hyperinflation. (Kindly provided by Dr Andrew Bush, Royal Brompton Hospital, London.)*

69

pneumothorax or pneumomediastinum. Bronchiectasis is often associated with asthmatic features, when the X-ray may show evidence of the underlying disease (see case 6, page 190). In children, unilateral wheeze may be associated with radiological features of foreign body aspiration, while in cystic fibrosis peribronchial thickening, atelectasis, consolidation or peripheral rounded abscesses may be seen.

Sinus X-rays and CT scans: Asthma is often associated with rhinitis, sinusitis or nasal polyps where changes may be seen on appropriate sinus X-rays. They are generally not advised in primary care investigations of patients. The views obtained by doctors are not always helpful and if a patient with suspected chronic sinusitis cannot be managed, referral for specialist advice is preferred. The ENT specialist may order a CT scan that will be more helpful than a sinus X-ray.

Blood tests: The differential white cell count may show eosinophilia in allergic asthma while the plasma viscosity or ESR are raised in Churge–Strauss syndrome and polyarteritis nodosa (both rare).

The total IgE level is elevated in cases of allergic asthma. Antigen-specific IgE can be detected using the radio-allergosorbent test (RAST) for allergens, including pollens, house dust mite, moulds, animal danders, *Aspergillus fumigatus* and food agents. The RAST test may be useful in evaluating certain occupational asthmas, e.g. bakers' asthma with positive levels to various flours, animal workers' asthma with raised levels to rats' urine protein, and in 20% of patients with isocyanate asthma. Serum IgE precipitins to *Aspergillus fumigatus* is found in 70% of cases of bronchopulmonary aspergillosis.

Skin allergy tests: An atopic constitution can be identified using skin prick testing with common inhaled allergens; the results sometimes influence management decisions (e.g. advice before purchasing bedding covers). There is a strong relationship between the positivity of skin tests to selected allergens and the levels of specific serum IgE. In asthma associated with the atopic state, a relationship exists between a history of specific allergic symptoms and the results of the skin tests. However, about 40% of normal individuals have positive reactions to common allergens and the results are often non-specific. A more accurate assessment of the clinical importance of inhaled allergens can be obtained from a detailed history. Positive tests may be useful in discussing the role of allergy with parents of children with asthma and rhinitis and, on occasions, may identify a single causative agent, e.g. cats and other household pets or laboratory animals, as the cause for asthma. A negative test to an allergen probably indicates it has little clinical significance. In very young children, skin tests are particularly unreliable.

The following tests are largely used in the research laboratory setting; however, they may occasionally be of use in clarifying a diagnosis.

Allergen challenge tests: Under strictly controlled conditions, in specialist hospital units, asthmatic patients may be exposed to increasing concentrations of inhaled allergens to establish the clinical importance of these agents or in clinical studies to demonstrate attenuation or blockage of the response by trial agents.

Provocation tests: Provocation tests may be used in the investigation of occupational asthma. The simplest test is to measure peak flow response following exposure to the agent in the working environment. More specific tests require the use of externally ventilated purpose-built provocation rooms to protect the investigators from exposure to the offending agents. Under these circumstances patients are exposed to small concentrations of the offending chemical and if sensitization exists a fall in the FEV_1 or peak flow will be observed.

Histamine and methacholine challenge tests: In the research laboratory, bronchial reactivity may be tested using aerosols of histamine and methacholine. The histamine or methacholine is generated as an aerosol via a nebulizer. Increasing, doubling concentrations are inhaled while changes in airway calibre are measured by serial FEV_1 readings which, when plotted against inhaled dosage on a logarithmic scale, produce a dose-response curve. The concentration of histamine or methacholine required to reduce the FEV_1 by 20% (PC_{20}) is a measure of airway responsiveness. The lower the PC_{20}, the greater the degree of airway hyperreactivity. Usually, a cumulative PC_{20} dose of <8 mg/ml histamine implies an individual has asthma and >8 mg/ml implies they do not (although the diagnosis is not completely excluded, especially if other clinical features in the history, examination and investigations suggest asthma). The test needs to be interpreted with caution in some individuals. Allergic rhinitics, who may not have obvious symptoms of asthma, may still have a PC_{20} <8 mg/ml histamine, which may be due to failure to recognise or variability of symptoms. For example, rhinitics with (or without) seasonal symptoms of asthma may have a PC_{20} <8 mg/ml during the season confirming a diagnosis of asthma, but >8 mg/ml when tested 'out of season' implying that the individual is non-asthmatic at the time. A fuller discussion of the pitfalls of using PC_{20} tests is to be found in Chapter 3.

Measurement of airways resistance: In the laboratory, airways resistance may be measured directly using the body plethysmograph but in practice this is largely a research tool.

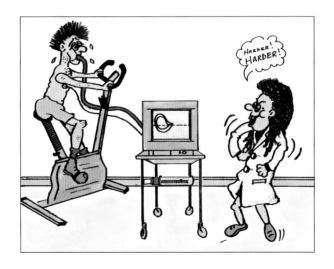

Improving the diagnosis of asthma: shared care

As discussed earlier in this chapter, many patients remain undiagnosed or experience long delays from the onset of symptoms to the diagnosis of asthma. The very nature of asthma, a chronic condition that relapses and remits, is a contributory factor to this delay because health professionals sometimes treat these patients as if they were suffering from a series of acute illnesses rather than one that is chronic. A major challenge is to heighten awareness, both for students as well as qualified health personnel, of the ways in which asthmatic patients present clinically. We think this is one of the shared tasks involving hospital as well as community health professionals.

The relapsing, remitting nature of asthma results in patients presenting themselves at different times and at different stages of their disease to different sectors of health-care provision. Good communication across the different sectors, of details of patient presentations with respiratory symptoms, may help to reduce the delay in diagnosing asthma.

There are five major sectors of health-care provision where potentially undiagnosed asthmatics may be identified. These are primary care, accident and emergency departments, medicine for the elderly, the school health services and health visitors.

Primary care

Having recognized those patients who present repeatedly with symptoms suggestive of asthma in primary care, health professionals may enhance their awareness and diagnosis of asthma by looking for clues in the medical records of patients and their families.

In the UK, patients' primary care NHS medical records contain information relating to consultations in all sectors of the service, for the duration of each individual's lifetime. These records of patients may be screened[4] in order to identify and recall possible undiagnosed asthmatics[6,21–24,42,43]. In one study[6], the author was able to increase the detected prevalence of diagnosed asthma by screening and subsequently recalling those children whose records had keywords suggestive of undiagnosed asthma. Neville's group[43] were able to demonstrate a beneficial clinical effect in those children who were identified as asthmatic by a trained facilitator and subsequently referred for treatment.

Accident and emergency (A&E) departments

For various reasons, some people use the A&E departments as their first port of call when ill. Undiagnosed asthmatic patients may form a substantial proportion of these and a concerted effort to identify them may enhance the individual's lifestyle through referral (usually to primary care) for appropriate treatment and may result in substantial health-care savings (through reduced A&E attendances and inappropriate use of antibiotics). Recurrent A&E attendances for asthma, i.e. within a few months, range from 12[44] to 17%[45]. Although the A&E department's main role is to deal with emergencies and to act as a filter for channelling patients appropriately in order to obtain treatment or advice, an additional role may be to identify repeat attenders, including those with diagnosed as well as undiagnosed asthma, and to try and reduce these numbers. This could be achieved by record-keeping systems that enable the staff to identify patients who have presented previously, e.g. computerized records using unique identifying fields, such as the patient's NHS number, with a brief summary of the dates and main reasons for attendance. In this way patients who use the A&E departments for obtaining repeat prescriptions (7% in one study[44] and 9% in another[45]) could be identified and then notified to their general practitioner who could make suitable arrangements for providing future repeat prescriptions. Similarly, the primary care team may be alerted (by a printout of attendances) when a patient with respiratory symptoms has attended the A&E department a number of times after surgery hours. Closer working relationships and enhanced communication between the A&E staff and those in primary care may be a way forward. After patients have been advised to contact their GP or practice nurse, follow-up telephone, fax or E-mail communication from the hospital could alert primary care members to a diagnosis of asthma or those individuals who are poorly controlled.

Medicine for the elderly

Many elderly asthmatic patients are undiagnosed; in fact, one study showed that there is a delay of over eight years in the diagnosis of asthma in patients over the age of 60 years[33]. An elderly patient complaining of respiratory symptoms may have asthma, chronic obstructive pulmonary disease or a combination of both. Investigation of this group of patients may be difficult if the person is unable to understand or perform PEF or spirometry tests. However, attempts to make a diagnosis should be made by the GP, as well as hospital outpatient staff and A&E departments. Sometimes exercise testing may be necessary as up to 15% of these patients may fail to perform adequate PEF or spirometry tests[25]. It is also worth reviewing the drug treatment in these patients as they may be taking medication such as beta blockers or non-steroidal anti-inflammatory drugs (NSAIDs) which could exacerbate asthma symptoms. If asthma is suspected and lung function tests are unhelpful, then a trial of therapy with inhaled or oral steroids may confirm the diagnosis. It would appear that published reports on underdiagnosis and the fact that most asthma deaths are in this age group, give weight to more attention being given to establishing a diagnosis in our elderly patients.

School health services and health visitors

Untapped resources in identifying undiagnosed asthmatics include health visitors who have a good knowledge of the medical and social background of the families of children in their care. They are well placed to recognize those children with recurrent respiratory symptoms; in the presence of risk factors for asthma diagnosis these children may be referred to the GP for further assessment. School nurses and doctors have a similar role to play in recognizing those undiagnosed asthmatic children who miss school repeatedly due to respiratory symptoms, and those who have difficulty in keeping up with their peers in sporting activities.

Making an early and accurate diagnosis is essential if the patient is to receive effective treatment. It is known that diagnosed asthmatic patients are treated more effectively than those who are not. When a diagnosis has been made, patients may be advised on measures to prevent as well as recognize attacks. They then have access to a wealth of information in books, magazines and through membership of patient-focused organizations such as the National Asthma Campaign in the UK. Thus applying the diagnostic label 'asthma' is preferable to the approach by many doctors who are reluctant to use the word asthma to explain the cause of their symptoms.

References

1 Godfrey S. Problems peculiar to the diagnosis and management of asthma in children. *BTTA Rev* 1974; **4**: 1–16.

2 Speight ANP. Is childhood asthma being underdiagnosed and undertreated? *BMJ* 1978; **2**: 331–2.

3 Speight ANP, Lee DA, Hey EN. Underdiagnosis and undertreatment of asthma in childhood. *Br Med J Clin Res Educ* 1983; **286**: 1253–6.

4 Levy M, Bell L. General practice audit of asthma in childhood. *Br Med J* 1984; **289**: 1115–16.

5 Levy M, Parmar M, Coetzee D, Duffy SW. Respiratory consultations in asthmatic compared with non-asthmatic children in general practice. *Br Med J* 1985; **291**: 29–30.

6 Heeijne Den Bak J. Prevalence and management of asthma in children under 16 in one practice. *BMJ* 1986; **292**: 175–6.

7 Anderson HR, Bailey PA, Cooper JS, Palmer JC, West S. Influence of morbidity illness label and social, family and health service factors on drug treatment of childhood asthma. *Lancet* 1981; **2**: 1030–2.

8 Wardman AG, Binns V, Clayden AD, Cooke NJ. The diagnosis and treatment of adults with obstructive airways disease in general practice. *Br J Dis Chest* 1986; **80**: 19–26.

9 Nish WA, Schweitz A. Underdiagnosis of asthma in young adults presenting for usaf basic training. *Ann Allergy* 1992; **69**: 239–42.

10 Hill R, Williams J, Britton J, Tattersfield A. Can morbidity associated with untreated asthma in primary schools be reduced?: A controlled intervention study. *BMJ* 1991; **303**: 1169–74.

11 Barnes PJ, Pedersen S. Efficacy and safety of inhaled corticosteroids in asthma. Report of a workshop held in Eze, France, October 1992. *Am Rev Respir Dis* 1993; **148**: S1–26.

12 Pedersen S. Clinical pharmacology and therapeutics. In: Silverman M, ed. *Childhood asthma and other wheezing disorders*. London: Chapman & Hall, 1995.

13 Djukanovic R, Roche WR, Wilson JW *et al.* Mucosal inflammation in asthma. *Am Rev Resp Dis* 1990; **142**: 434–57.

14 Strachan DP. Epidemiology. In: Silverman M, ed. *Childhood asthma and other wheezing disorders.* London: Chapman & Hall, 1995.

15 The British Thoracic Society, The National Asthma Campaign, The Royal College of Physicians of London *et al.* The British guidelines on asthma management: 1995 Review and position statement. *Thorax* 1997; **52**(Suppl.): S1–21.

16 Jones A, Sykes AP. The effect of symptom presentation on delay in asthma diagnosis in children in a general practice. *Resp Med* 1990; **84**: 139–42.

17 Tudor-Hart J. Wheezing in young children: problems of measurement and management. *J Roy Coll Gen Pract* 1986; **36**: 78–81.

18 Charlton I, Jones K, Bain J. Delay in diagnosis of childhood asthma and its influence on respiratory consultation rates. *Arch Dis Childh* 1991; **66**: 633–5.

19 Levy M. Royal College of General Practitioners Audit Programme — Asthma Audit: two recommendations for general practice. *Eur Resp J* 1994; **7**(Suppl. 18): 915.

20 Levy ML, Barnes GR, Howe M, Neville RG. Provision of primary care asthma services in the United Kingdom. *Thorax* 1996; **51**: A28.

21 Levy M. Delay in diagnosing asthma — is the nature of general practice to blame? [editorial]. *J Roy Coll Gen Pract* 1986; **36**: 52–3.

22 Levy ML, Hilton SR. *Asthma in practice.* London: Royal College of General Practitioners, 1993.

23 Levy ML. Primary care. In: O'Byrne PO, Thomson NC, eds. *Manual of asthma management.* London, Philadelphia, Toronto, Sydney, Tokyo: W.B. Saunders Co. Ltd. 1995; 767–90.

24 Toop LJ. Active approach to recognising asthma in general practice. *BMJ* 1985; **290**: 1629–31.

25 Dow L. The diagnosis of asthma in older people. *Clin Exp Allergy* 1994; **24**: 156–9.

26 Doan T, Patterson R, Greenberger PA. Cough variant asthma: usefulness of a diagnostic-therapeutic trial with prednisone *Ann Allergy* 1992; **69**: 505–9.

27 Johnson D, Osborn LM. Cough variant asthma: a review of the clinical literature. *J Asthma* 1991; **28**: 85–90.

28 Boggs PB. Asthma and bronchitis. *J Allergy Clin Immunol* 1993; **84**: 1055–8.

29 Orr AW. Prodromal itching in asthma. *J Roy Coll Gen Pract* 1979; **29**: 287–8.

30 David TJ, Wybrew M, Hennessen U. Prodromal itching in childhood asthma. *Lancet* 1984; **21**: 154–5.

31 Burge PS. Occupational and environmental asthma. In: Clark TJH, Godfrey S, Lee TH, eds. *Asthma.* London, New York, Tokyo, Melbourne, Madras: Chapman & Hall, 1992; 308–40.

32 Burge PS. Single and serial measurements of lung function in the diagnosis of occupational asthma. *Eur J Resp Dis* 1982; **63**: 47–59.

33 Dow L. The epidemiology and therapy of airflow limitation in the elderly. *Drugs and Ageing* 1992; **2**: 546–59.

34 Jones PW. Quality of life, symptoms and pulmonary function in asthma: long-term treatment with nedocromil sodium examined in a controlled multicentre trial. Nedocromil sodium quality of life study group. *Eur Resp J* 1994; **7**: 55–62.

35 Jones PW, Quirke FH, Bavestock CM, Littlejohns P. A self complete measure of health status for chronic airflow limitation. The St. George's respiratory questionnaire. *Am Rev Resp Dis* 1992; **145**: 1321–7.

36 Hyland ME, Crocker GR. Validation of an asthma quality of life diary in a clinical trial. *Thorax* 1995; **50**: 724–30.

37 Juniper EF, Johnston PR, Borkhoff CM *et al.* Quality of life in asthma clinical trials: comparison of salmeterol and salbutamol. *Am J Resp Crit Care Med* 1995; **151**: 66–70.

38 Juniper EF, Guyatt GH, Willan A, Griffith LE. Determining a minimal important change in a disease-specific quality of life questionnaire. *J Clin Epidemiol* 1994; **47**: 81–7.

39 Juniper EF, Guyatt GH, Ferrie PJ, Griffith LE. Measuring quality of life in asthma. *Am Rev Resp Dis* 1993; **147**: 832–8.

40 Juniper EF, Guyatt GH, Epstein RS, Ferrie PJ, Jaeschke R, Hiller TK. Evaluation of impairment of health related quality of life in asthma: development of a questionnaire for use in clinical trials. *Thorax* 1992; **47**: 76–83.

41 Department of Health. *Drug tariff* London: HMSO, 1996.

42 Neville RG, Bryce FP, Robertson FM, Crombie IK, Clark RA. Diagnosis and treatment of asthma in children: usefulness of a review of medical records. *Br J Gen Pract* 1992; **42**: 501–3.

43 Bryce FP, Neville RG, Crombie IK, Clark RA, McKenzie P. Controlled trial of an audit facilitator in diagnosis and treatment of childhood asthma in general practice. *BMJ* 1995; **310**: 838–42.

44 Partridge MR, Latouche D, Trako E, Thurston JB. A national census of those attending UK accident and emergency departments with asthma. *J Acc Emerg Med* 1977; **14**: 16–20.

45 Levy M, Robb M, Bradley J, Winter R. Patient self-management of acute asthma: a prospective study in two districts. *Clin Sci* 1993; **84**: (Suppl. 28), 39p.

Chapter 5

Management

Principles of effective management

The main aims of management in asthma are to:

- abolish symptoms
- maintain best possible lung function
- reduce the frequency and severity of acute episodes
- minimize incapacity such as time lost off school or work.

These aims should be achieved with as little medication and disruption of the patient's and their family's lives as possible. They are best met by a partnership between patients, their families and health professionals (primary, secondary or tertiary health-care teams). Good communication is essential. To be effective, sufficient time has to be set aside to discuss the principles of management followed by review visits for reinforcement[1,2].

The patient's concerns and fears, and the particular needs of adolescents, the unemployed and the elderly need to be appropriately addressed. The patient/parent needs to be actively involved in the development of management plans; the objective is to empower the patient to manage their own asthma effectively and safely. Although initially time consuming, these efforts will be rewarded in the longer term by better asthma control, improved quality of life for the patients and less emergency contact with health-care professionals[3].

The rational use of drugs effective in relieving and preventing asthma symptoms should include an appropriate device for the person's age, aptitude and ability. Regular assessment, adjustment of medication and follow-up are very important. Prevention is always better than cure; therefore identification and avoidance, where possible, of trigger factors that may significantly reduce symptoms is the logical starting point.

Avoidance of trigger factors

While one particular trigger, e.g. allergy or infection, may initiate the development of asthma in an individual, once the process has become established any other trigger may act to reinforce the inflammatory process, thereby perpetuating the inflammation in the bronchial walls (Figure 5.1). The relative importance of the various trigger factors in producing symptoms may vary during a patient's lifetime. Thus, in childhood, allergies may be a major factor, whereas in adult life infection may predominate. The terms *extrinsic asthma*, referring to wheeze predominantly precipitated by environmental factors such as allergy and inhaled irritants, and *intrinsic asthma*, where the major factors are not identifiable, have been used to describe the nature of an individual with asthma. They are difficult to distinguish in clinical practice, and a more pragmatic approach is to consider asthma as a common response to different insults, some intrinsic and some extrinsic.

A knowledge of the common allergens that trigger wheezy episodes is important but can be difficult to establish (see boxes).

Pets: A careful history and sometimes home visits may be necessary to establish which particular trigger is responsible. At times these may be unusual: a newsagent developed an allergy to maggots that he was rearing to sell to local fishermen! Many schools now have furry animals in the classroom. An allergic child may well develop an allergy to a new pet after a few months; therefore, parents of children with asthma and other atopic diseases should be advised not to buy pets. Cats and dogs should not be allowed into the bedroom or living room, where children spend a lot of time playing on the floor. Frequent bathing or damp-washing of cats and dogs can reduce symptoms by reducing exposure to their allergens.

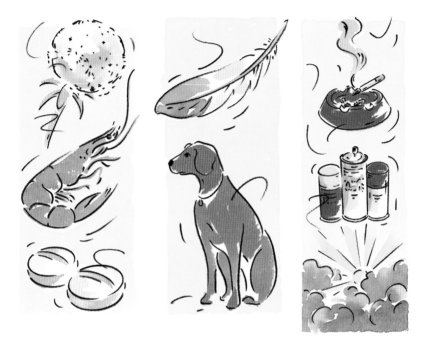

Figure 5.1 *Avoidable trigger factors. (Reproduced with permission from Glaxo Wellcome UK Ltd.)*

Potential trigger factors for adult asthma attacks

- Pollution (smoking indoors, outdoors)
- Drugs
- Pollen (tree, grass)
- Alcohol
- Foods (shellfish, peanuts)
- Aerosols/perfumes
- Preservatives(sulphur dioxide)
- Food colouring (E102, tartrazine)
- Occupation (e.g. spray paints)
- Cold temperature

> **Potential trigger factors for childhood asthma attacks**
>
> ■ Viral infections
> ■ Exercise
> ■ Allergen exposure
> ■ Cigarette smoke
> ■ Emotional upset
> ■ Chemical irritants
> ■ Cold air.

Exposure to pets may not always be in the home: visits to friends and relatives, and leisure pursuits such as horse riding may exacerbate attacks.

Smoking: Involuntary (passive) smoking adversely affects many people with asthma[4] imposing limitations on their leisure activities: they may have to leave discotheques, pubs and other social events owing to the effects of a smoky environment. Between a third and a half of asthmatic children in Britain live in a home where at least one adult smokes. The more cigarettes the adult smokes, the greater the effect on the child. Maternal smoking seems to be more important than paternal smoking, because of increased exposure; infants are more susceptible than older children[5].

Children with asthma are particularly sensitive to tobacco smoke in that they have:

■ more frequent and severe symptoms
■ an earlier onset of asthma
■ greater use of asthma medications
■ worse lung function
■ more frequent respiratory infections, such as bronchiolitis and pneumonia.

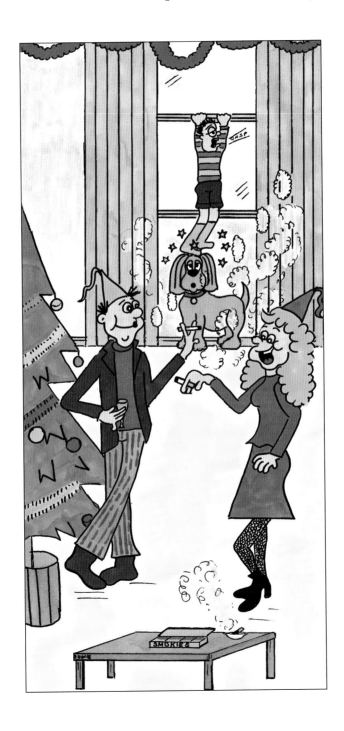

Maternal smoking in pregnancy has effects on the fetus and neonate, including:

■ impaired lung development

■ smaller and more reactive airways

■ repeated wheeze, cough and breathlessness in the first few years of life, particularly if there is a family history of atopic disease.

As 38% of women in this country smoke regularly in early pregnancy, the implications of these findings are serious.

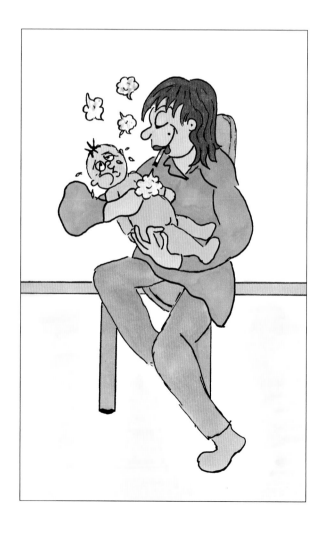

An employee with asthma working in an open office where smoking is permitted, or having to use a smoky rest room, may be badly affected. They may need to seek alternative employment unless their working environment is changed. Employees may be liable for compensation if this occurs.

House dust mite: Many asthmatic children have evidence of allergy to the house dust mite. There has been a marked rise in house dust mite concentrations in modern centrally heated, double-glazed, poorly ventilated homes that form an ideal breeding ground. Regular hoovering of the carpets and bed, damp-dusting of the woodwork and regular washing and changing of the bedding should be encouraged; the benefits of ionizers, humidifiers and acaricides remain unproven.

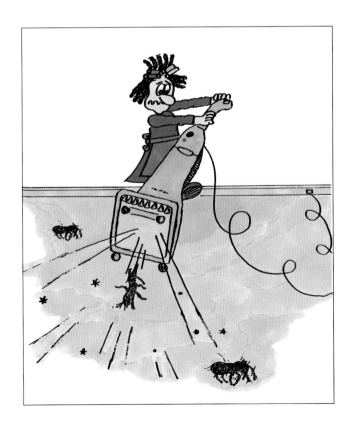

Food and drink: Food allergies are rarely a major cause of wheezing episodes in children or adults, although the colouring agent tartrazine in some children's drinks and desserts, cooking oils, shellfish and strawberries should be avoided if they are shown to be implicated[7]. Very occasionally severe anaphylactic reactions may follow the ingestion of nuts, mustard and meat extracts inadvertently taken in a restaurant. Anyone who is allergic to nuts needs to be very aware that nut oil (peanut, groundnut) is sometimes used to prepare fish and chips and other fast foods; these individuals may need to carry a loaded adrenaline syringe for emergency use.

A small number of asthmatic patients react after drinking alcoholic beverages, usually those with a heavy sediment, such as beers and red wines, but a 'safe' alternative can usually be found[8].

Occupational hazards: Some patients may develop occupational asthma as a result of being exposed to respiratory sensitizers in the workplace (see Table 5.1). Sensitizers recognized by the DSS (UK) for compensation include: dusts from insects, animals and products containing them; dust from tea, beans and wood; flour, grain and hay; and glues, resins, soldering fumes and chemicals.

Anyone with suspected occupational asthma should be referred to a physician with a special interest in this field. Affected workers should seek redeployment in a 'safe' working area and only as a last resort change their jobs.

Drug reactions: While not all asthmatic adults react adversely to aspirin and non-steroidal anti-inflammatory drugs (NSAIDs), care needs to be taken when prescribing them as reactions can be swift and severe[9]. One should always check medications prescribed for other concomitant diseases, such as hypertension, angina and glaucoma, as the prescription of drugs such as beta blockers may adversely affect asthma control. Similar drug reactions are very uncommon in children with asthma.

Table 5.1 Agents causing asthma in selected occupations[11]

Occupation/ Occupational field	Agent
Miscellaneous	
Laboratory animal workers/vets	Dander and urine proteins
Food processing	Shellfish, egg proteins, pancreatic enzymes, papain, amylase
Dairy farmers	Storage mites
Poultry farmers	Poultry mites, droppings and feathers
Granary workers	Storage mites, *Aspergillus*, indoor ragweed and grass pollen
Research workers	Locusts
Fish food manufacturing	Midges
Detergent manufacturing	*Bacillus subtilis* enzymes
Silk workers	Silk-worm moths and larvae
Plant proteins	
Bakers	Flour, amylase
Food processing	Coffee bean dust, meat tenderizer (papain), tea
Farmers	Soy bean dust
Shipping workers	Grain dust (moulds, insects, grain)
Laxative manufacturing	Ispaghula, psyllium
Sawmill workers, carpenters	Wood dust (Western red cedar, oak, mahogany, zebrawood, red wood, Lebanon cedar, African maple, Eastern white cedar)
Electric soldering	Colophony (pine resin)
Cotton textile workers	Cotton dust
Nurses	Psyllium, latex

Table 5.1 (contd.)

Inorganic chemicals

Refinery workers	Platinum salts, vanadium
Plating	Nickel salts
Diamond polishing	Cobalt salts
Manufacturing	Aluminium fluoride
Beauty shop	Persulfate
Welding	Stainless steel fumes, chromium salts

Organic chemicals

Manufacturing	Antibiotics, piperazine, methyl dopa, salbutamol, cimetidine
Hospital workers	Disinfectants (sulfathiazole, chloramine, formaldehyde, glutaraldehyde)
Anaesthesiology	Enflurane
Poultry workers	Aprolium
Fur dyeing	Paraphenylene diamine
Rubber processing	Formaldehyde, ethylene diamine, phthalic anhydride
Plastics industry	Toluene diisocyanate, hexamethyl diisocyanate, diphenylmethyl isocyanate, phthalic anhydride, triethylene tetramines, trimellitic anhydride, hexamethyl tetramine
Automobile painting	Dimethyl ethanolamine diisocyanate
Foundry worker	Reaction product of furan binder

Rhinitis

Asthma and rhinitis often coexist: over 65% of children attending a paediatric respiratory clinic have been found to have symptoms such as mouth breathing, snoring or persistent nasal stuffiness, suggesting significant rhinitis (unpublished audit). As a result of nasal obstruction, air inhaled through the mouth gets direct unfiltered access to the bronchial tree and this can increase the harmful effects of irritants and allergens. In addition, rhinitis may account for nocturnal cough which is unresponsive to increasing asthma medication. When this problem is treated vigorously with antihistamines or topical nasal steroids, the nasal symptoms may be relieved and asthma control improved, allowing a reduction in the dose of prophylactic asthma medication.

People who complain of exacerbations of symptoms under specific circumstances such as visiting a relative who has a dog, could be advised to double up their prophylactic medication and take their bronchodilators regularly two or three days before, during and after the visit. Similarly, it is generally recommended that the patients should double their prophylactic medication and take their bronchodilators regularly at the onset of a cold until cold symptoms settle.

Drug therapy

There are three main categories of drugs used in the management of asthma: preventers, relievers and emergency drugs, as shown in the box.

Preventers

Drugs in this group act by blocking the release and action of the mediators from mast cells, nerves and other cells involved in the inflammatory response in the bronchial mucosa (sodium cromoglycate, nedocromil sodium) or by suppressing the inflammation (corticosteroids), thereby reducing the bronchial hyperreactivity or 'twitchiness' of the bronchi. The more reactive the airway, the smaller the trigger needed to produce a wheezy episode. The production of British and International asthma treatment guidelines have been a major step in rationalizing the use of preventative or prophylactic medication[1,2,10–14].

Categories of drugs used in asthma management

Preventers
- mast cell stabilizers
- inhaled corticosteroids
- ? theophyllines
- ? leukotriene antagonists
- systemic steroids

Relievers
- beta-2-adrenergic bronchodilators (short-acting/long-acting)
- antimuscarinics
- theophyllines

Emergency drugs
- systemic steroids
- high-dose bronchodilators
- oxygen

The preventers form the mainstay of modern asthma treatment. Any patient who needs to use inhaled bronchodilators on a daily basis should be on prophylactic medication[10]. To be effective, prophylactic medication must be taken regularly. Twice daily regimes give better compliance and improved control compared with more frequent administrations[15]. It is important that patients and parents are informed at the onset that although the medication will start working straight away, the full effect may not be obvious for several weeks. Failure to do this often leads to problems if patients discontinue their medication, making it more difficult to stabilize their asthma.

A further problem occurs when patients do not adhere to medical advice: their asthma fails to resolve and their symptoms may get worse.

Over recent years there has been a dramatic increase in prescription numbers for inhaled steroids for asthma; they rose from

1.13 million in 1980 to 8.53 million per annum in 1993. A practice that takes an active interest in asthma management tends to prescribe a high proportion of prophylactic medication[16]. There is good evidence that in many areas appropriate assessment and management of asthma is still not ideal and it is likely that the use of prophylactic medication will continue to increase in the future.

Mast cell stabilizers: For many years sodium cromoglycate was the most widely used preventative treatment in children with frequent mild to moderate symptoms. However, with the increasing evidence of greater efficacy of inhaled steroids and reassuring safety data about inhaled steroids in conventional doses, many clinicians now regard low-dose inhaled steroids as their first-line preventative therapy in children. This shift in practice is reflected in the new revised British guidelines[10]. In adults, nedocromil sodium may be helpful for those patients who experience adverse effects from inhaled steroids and those who suffer from troublesome cough due to their asthma (see page 115).

Inhaled corticosteroids: The introduction of inhaled corticosteroids in the late 1960s revolutionized the management of chronic asthma and they are now established as the mainstay of prophylactic medication. Inhaled corticosteroids are the most effective preventative drugs we have for asthma in children and adults. Whether our aim is to control symptoms, to reduce airway hyper-reactivity, or to suppress bronchial inflammation, inhaled steroids are the standard by which other preventers are judged.

Inhaled corticosteroids, are safer than **regular** oral corticosteroids which have many adverse effects:

- osteoporosis
- diabetes
- hypertension
- cushingoid features
- obesity
- infection

91

- avascular necrosis of the femoral head
- adrenal suppression.

Fortunately, these complications are seen rarely since the introduction of inhaled steroids[17].

In adults prescribed daily doses of <800 µg beclomethasone dipropionate or budesonide, and 400 µg of fluticasone propionate, there is little evidence of any biochemical or clinically important systemic corticosteroid effects, although there may be some local problems in the throat such as dysphonia and/or thrush[16].

There are currently three inhaled steroids available on prescription in the UK: beclomethasone dipropionate (BDP) (Becotide, Aerobec, Filair, Becloforte), budesonide (Pulmicort) and fluticasone propionate (Flixotide). All have potent, complex anti-inflammatory effects on the bronchial mucosa. They differ in their pharmacodynamic properties, such as their absorption, their binding to lung receptors and their metabolism. Beclomethasone dipropionate and budesonide are of equal clinical potency while fluticasone propionate is twice as potent[18,19]. However, current evidence suggests that the risk/benefit ratio for fluticasone and budesonide are similar at equipotent doses but the inhaler device used is an important determinant of systemic activity. All inhaled steroids can produce biochemical abnormalities when used in high doses.

The potential side effects of inhaled steroids can be divided into local and systemic effects. **Local effects** are due to drug deposition in the mouth and throat. Candidiasis is much less common in children than in adults[18,20]. The incidence is less with spacers or dry powder inhalers than with pressurized metered dose inhalers[19,20]. Mouth-washing or tooth-brushing after inhalation further reduces the risk. Dysphonia, an effect on the laryngeal muscles, is also uncommon: it usually resolves if the drug is stopped[18,20].

The potential **systemic effects** of inhaled steroids are due to absorption into the circulation. Many factors influence absorption. It was originally thought that the 80–90% of an inhaled dose that is swallowed and absorbed from the gastrointestinal tract led to systemic effects. As fluticasone propionate has the lowest oral bioavailability, it was thought it would have less systemic activity. It is now accepted that there is also absorption of the 10–20% of the inhaled dose which enters the lung: this is similar for all three drugs[18]. Efficient inhalers that deliver a high dose to the lungs increase systemic absorption[21]. This is clinically relevant: for example, if children are changed from receiving budesonide via a Nebuhaler to via a Turbohaler, which gives better lung deposition, the dose can be halved for the same therapeutic effect[21,22]. Inhaler technique also influences absorption but dosage has the biggest influence — the bigger the dose, the greater absorption and the potential for side effects.

The important potential systemic side effects of inhaled steroids are on the adrenal gland, bone and growth. At high doses, all three drugs produce biochemical evidence of **adrenocortical suppression**. This effect is dose-related: for the conventional doses (200–400 µg/day of BDP or budesonide, or half that dose of fluticasone) that control symptoms well in most children, any minor effect is not significant[18,20].

Theoretically, long-term inhaled steroid therapy may affect **bone turnover** leading to osteoporosis. In certain at-risk adults, such as postmenopausal women, concern may be appropriate. In children, inhaled steroids do affect chemical markers of bone turnover at high doses, but children, who have taken 400–800 µg/day of inhaled steroids for many years, have normal bone density and no evidence of osteoporosis[23].

Assessing the **effects on growth** is more difficult. Moderate or severe asthma in itself can delay growth and puberty, although normal adult height is eventually achieved. Several studies have shown a dose-related reduction in short-term leg growth with 400–800 µg/day of inhaled steroids: BDP had a greater effect than budesonide or fluticasone[18,20]. The significance of these findings is unclear as most long-term studies have shown normal growth in children on inhaled steroids[23]. Indeed, the better symptom control they produce may improve growth.

Parents can be reassured that inhaled steroids produce no significant side effects at the doses most children need[18,20]. Once control is achieved, it is often possible to reduce the dose. The most appropriate inhaler device should be selected on the basis of a child's age, aptitude and ability. If normal doses fail to give good control, the addition of another drug may be considered, such as salmeterol or eformoterol, rather than the automatic doubling of the steroid dose. In children on all but the lowest doses of an inhaled steroid, height should be measured and charted accurately every six months, so that any effect on growth is identified promptly.

Antileukotriene therapy: Oral agents that block the broncho-constrictor and other actions of leukotrienes, potent mediators released from mast cells and eosinophils, will soon be available in the UK. Their exact place in long-term management of adults and children is currently being evaluated. They are of particular value in adults with aspirin-sensitive asthma[24].

Oral steroids and immunosuppressant agents: There are a few patients who still require a small daily dose of oral steroids to control their symptoms despite the use of inhaled steroids and long-acting bronchodilators.

Before such management is started, it is essential that:

■ The patient's lifestyle is checked to control trigger factors, such as exposure to pets or environmental tobacco smoke

■ Therapy using inhaled corticosteroids and oral and inhaled bronchodilators, theophyllines and mast cell stabilizers is optimized so as to ensure that the dose of oral steroids required is as low as possible.

Advice from a specialist is advisable in those patients who require continuous oral corticosteroid therapy. Very few children with asthma require continuous therapy with oral corticosteroids. Those that do should be referred to a paediatric respiratory specialist because children are particularly susceptible to the adverse effects of oral steroids, most notably the suppression of normal growth. Children who need continuous oral steroid therapy are usually prescribed an alternate morning regime as this has the least suppressant effect on growth.

A number of immunosuppressant agents, e.g. methotrexate, cyclophosphamide and cyclosporin, have been tried in the management of difficult cases of adult asthma, at times successfully. These patients should be managed by the hospital service. These drugs have no place in the management of childhood asthma.

Relievers

These drugs produce bronchodilation by relaxing the bronchial smooth muscle. They have little effect on the underlying inflammatory reaction and are principally used to relieve wheezy episodes.

Short-acting beta-2 agonists: While inhalers are the delivery system of choice, oral preparations are available for young children, but are of lesser efficacy, and should be used only in children unable to take the drugs by inhalation. Oral beta-2 agonists may cause tremor and anxiety in a child.

The commonly used short acting beta-2 agonists are salbutamol and terbutaline which produce bronchodilation within minutes and have an action of 4–6 hours. Beta-2 agonists taken before sport or regularly at the onset of an upper respiratory tract infection can help to prevent exercise-induced symptoms or an exacerbation of asthma associated with colds. Side effects are less common in children than adults. If one drug produces tremors, tachycardia or arrhythmias, the alternative could be tried as the action is often drug specific.

Long-acting beta-2 agonists: The long-acting beta-2 agonists, salmeterol and eformoterol, have a duration of action lasting 12–18 hours. Their main indications are to control nocturnal and exercise-induced symptoms that persist despite adequate doses of inhaled steroids[25]. They are **not** a replacement for inhaled steroids (i.e. they should not be used alone) as they have little or no anti-inflammatory action and should be used only in children and adults who are already taking inhaled topical steroids. They bind tightly to beta-2 receptors and it is potentially dangerous to take them together with **regular** short-acting beta-2 agonists, mainly because the patient loses the important early warning system provided by their need for extra relief medication. They have a slower onset of action than short-acting beta-2 agonists and should not be used for acute relief of wheezy episodes. The advice on long-acting beta-2 agonists has recently changed in the revised British Guidelines[10].

Slow-release oral preparations of beta-2 agonists are available for patients who cannot use inhalers or require oral therapy. They are rarely used in children.

Anticholinergic drugs: The anticholinergic (antimuscarinic) drugs ipratropium bromide (Atrovent) and oxytropium bromide (Oxivent) produce bronchodilation by blocking the effects of acetylcholine released at vagal bronchoconstrictor nerve endings. These drugs may be used as an alternative to beta-2 agonists in adult patients who develop unacceptable side effects such as tremor. They complement the action of beta-2 agonists and are commonly used in combination with them in severe forms of asthma[26]. Maximum bronchodilation occurs after 30–40 minutes and lasts 4–6 hours with ipratropium or 12 hours with oxytropium. They are of limited value in the management of children, but may be effective in acute wheezing episodes in children in the first 12–18 months of life.

Theophyllines: Theophyllines act through inhibiting the cyclic nucleotide phosphodiesterase pathways to produce bronchodilation. They have a narrow therapeutic range which necessitates monitoring serum levels if the maximum effect is to be observed with the least possible risk of side effects. This limits their use in general practice and in hospital care. A number of patients develop side effects that may be due to the action both locally (the stomach) and in the central nervous system (nausea, vomiting, restlessness and confusion) or, in adults, on the cardiovascular system with arrhythmias and hypertension. Controlled-release oral preparations are useful for twice daily regimes in adults. The high incidence of side effects in children, and the appearance of more effective inhaled therapy over the last 12–15 years, has led to a marked decline in their use in children.

Clinical, histological and cellular evidence is accumulating that suggests that theophyllines have at least an anti-inflammatory as well as a bronchodilator effect. This action has been noted at a relatively low dose where side effects are less likely to be a problem[27]. If other studies confirm their anti-inflammatory role, the theophyllines may have a beneficial steroid-sparing effect in adults. There is no evidence that these effects are present in children with asthma. Clinical trials are being undertaken on other inhibitors of the cyclic nucleotide phosphodiesterases where the effects are greater on the inflammatory component.

Emergency drugs

Asthma still claims the lives of too many young people[28,29]. One possible explanation may be that in acute exacerbations of asthma, systemic steroids are still underused. Any patient with an acute asthma attack must be assessed properly and treated aggressively[1,2,10,30]. The treatment of acute attacks and the drugs and dosages are shown in Figure 5.2.

Oral or intravenous steroids should be given early and in an effective dose, the duration of treatment depending on the response. The use of PEF charts during acute exacerbations of asthma is a logical way to determine when the attack has ended and therefore when the oral steroid therapy can safely be discontinued. The course may be stopped abruptly. It is rarely necessary to tail the dose off, unless patients are discontinuing a long-term continuous course of oral steroids. Any adult patient receiving systemic steroids for an acute asthma attack should be either started on prophylactic inhaled steroids or have their dose increased until 3 months after their symptoms have settled and lung function has returned to normal. An acute exacerbation of asthma often originates from inadequate maintenance therapy.

Chart 2

Acute severe asthma in adults

Recognition and assessment in hospital

Features of acute severe asthma

- Peak expiratory flow (PEF) ≤ 50% of predicted or best
- Can't complete sentences in one breath
- Respirations ≥ 25 breaths/min
- Pulse > 110 beats/min

Life threatening features

- PEF < 33% of predicted or best
- Silent chest, cyanosis, or feeble respiratory effort
- Bradycardia or hypotension
- Exhaustion, confusion, or coma

If SaO_2 < 92% or a patient has **any life threatening** features, measure arterial blood gases.

Blood gas markers of a very severe, life threatening attack:

- Normal (5–6 kPa, 36–45 mm Hg) or high $PaCO_2$
- Severe hypoxia: PaO_2 < 8 kPa (60 mm Hg) irrespective of treatment with oxygen
- A low pH (or high H+)

No other investigations are needed for immediate management.

Caution
Patients with severe or life threatening attacks may not be distressed and may not have all these abnormalities. The presence of any should alert the doctor

---

1 Immediate treatment

- Oxygen 40–60% (CO_2 retention is not usually aggravated by oxygen therapy in asthma)
- Salbutamol 5 mg or terbutaline 10 mg via an oxygen driven nebuliser
- Prednisolone tablets 30–60 mg or intravenous hydrocortisone 200 mg or both if very ill
- No sedatives of any kind
- Chest radiograph to exclude pneumothorax

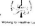
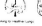

Peak expiratory flow in normal adults

From Gregg I, Nunn AJ. BMJ 1989; 298: 1068–70

IF LIFE THREATENING FEATURES ARE PRESENT:

- Add ipratropium 0.5 mg to the nebulised β agonist
- Give intravenous aminophylline 250 mg over 20 minutes or salbutamol or terbutaline 250 µg over 10 minutes. Do not give bolus aminophylline to patients already taking oral theophyllines

2 Subsequent management

IF PATIENT IS IMPROVING CONTINUE:

- 40–60% oxygen
- Prednisolone 30–60 mg daily or intravenous hydrocortisone 200 mg 6 hourly
- Nebulised β agonist 4 hourly

IF PATIENT IS NOT IMPROVING AFTER 15–30 MINUTES:

- Continue oxygen and steroids
- Give nebulised β agonist more frequently, up to every 15–30 minutes
- Add ipratropium 0.5 mg to nebuliser and repeat 6 hourly until patient is improving

IF PATIENT IS STILL NOT IMPROVING GIVE:

- Aminophylline infusion (small patient 750 mg/24 hours, large patient 1500 mg/24 hours); monitor blood concentrations if it is continued for over 24 hours
- Salbutamol or terbutaline infusion as an alternative to aminophylline

3 Monitoring treatment

- Repeat measurement of PEF 15–30 minutes after starting treatment
- Oximetry: maintain SaO_2 > 92%
- Repeat blood gas measurements within 2 hours of starting treatment if

- initial PaO_2 < 8 kPa (60 mmHg) unless subsequent SaO_2 > 92%
- $PaCO_2$ normal or raised patient deteriorates
- Chart PEF before and after giving nebulised or inhaled β agonists and at least 4 times daily throughout hospital stay

Transfer patient to the intensive care unit accompanied by a doctor prepared to intubate if there is:

- Deteriorating PEF, worsening or persisting hypoxia, or hypercapnia
- Exhaustion, feeble respirations, confusion or drowsiness
- Coma or respiratory arrest

4 When discharged from hospital, patients should have:

- Been on discharge medication for 24 hours and *have had inhaler technique checked and recorded*
- PEF > 75% of predicted or best and PEF diurnal variability < 25% *unless discharge is agreed with respiratory physician*
- Treatment with *oral and inhaled steroids* in addition to brochodilators
- Own PEF meter and *written self management plan*
- GP follow up arranged *within 1 week*
- Follow up appointment in respiratory clinic *within 4 weeks*

Also

- Determine reason(s) for exacerbation and admission
- Send details of admission, discharge and potential best PEF to GP

Adapted from poster designed by Business Design Group

NATIONAL ASTHMA CAMPAIGN
Working for Healthier Lungs

In association with the General Practitioner in Asthma Group, the British Association of Accident and Emergency Medicine, the British Paediatric Respiratory Society and the Royal College of Paediatrics and Child Health

---

Figure 5.2 *Selected charts from the British guidelines in asthma management[10]. (Reproduced by permission from BMJ Publications.). Continued overleaf.*

Chart 3

Acute severe asthma
in those aged 5–15 years

Recognition of acute severe asthma

- Too breathless to talk
- Too breathless to feed
- Respirations ≥ 40 breaths/min
- Pulse ≥ 120 beats/min
- PEF ≤ 50% predicted or best

No other investigations are needed for immediate management

Blood gas estimations are rarely helpful in deciding initial management in children

Life threatening features

- PEF < 33% predicted or best
- Cyanosis, silent chest, or poor respiratory effort
- Fatigue or exhaustion
- Agitation or reduced level of consciousness

Caution:
Children with severe attacks may not appear distressed; assessment in the very young may be difficult. The presence of any of these features should alert the doctor.

Management of a severe asthma attack

1 Immediate treatment

- High flow oxygen via face mask
- Salbutamol 5 mg or terbutaline 10 mg via an oxygen driven nebuliser (half doses in very young children)
- Prednisolone 1–2 mg/kg body weight orally (maximum 40 mg)

IF LIFE THREATENING FEATURES ARE PRESENT:

- Give intravenous aminophylline 5 mg/kg over 20 minutes followed by maintenance infusion, 1 mg/kg/h; omit the loading dose if child already receiving oral theophyllines

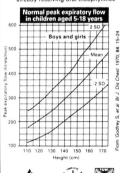

Normal peak expiratory flow in children aged 5–18 years

Boys and girls

Mean

+2 SD

−2 SD

Peak expiratory flow (litres/min)

600
500
400
300
200
100

Height (cm)
110 120 130 140 150 160 170

From: Godfrey S, et al Br J Dis Chest 1970; 64 15–24

 NATIONAL ASTHMA CAMPAIGN
campaigning together

Working for Healthier Lungs

- Give intravenous hydrocortisone 100 mg 6 hourly
- Add ipratropium 0.25 mg to nebulised β agonist (0.125 mg in very young children)
- Pulse oximetry is helpful in assessing response to treatment. An Sao₂ ≤ 92% may indicate the need for chest radiography.

2 Subsequent management

IF PATIENT IS IMPROVING CONTINUE:

- High flow oxygen
- Prednisolone 1–2 mg/kg daily (maximum 40 mg/day)
- Nebulised β agonist 4 hourly

IF PATIENT IS NOT IMPROVING AFTER 15–30 MINUTES:

- Continue oxygen and steroids
- Give nebulised β agonist more frequently, up to every 30 minutes
- Add ipratropium to nebuliser and repeat 6 hourly until improvement starts

IF PATIENT IS STILL NOT IMPROVING GIVE:

- Aminophylline infusion (1 mg/kg/h); monitor blood concentrations if continued for over 24 hours

3 Monitoring treatment

- Repeat PEF measurement 15–30 minutes after starting treatment (if appropriate)
- Oximetry: maintain Sao₂ > 92%
- Chart PEF if appropriate before and after the child inhales β agonists and at least 4 times daily throughout hospital stay

4 Transfer to the intensive care unit accompanied by a doctor prepared to intubate if there is:

- Deteriorating PEF, worsening or persisting hypoxia, or hypercapnia
- Exhaustion, feeble respirations, confusion or drowsiness
- Coma or respiratory arrest

5 When discharged from hospital patients should have:

- Been on discharge medication for 24 hours and have had inhaler technique checked and recorded
- If recorded, PEF > 75% of predicted or best and PEF diurnal variability < 25%
- Treatment with soluble steroid tablets and inhaled steroids in addition to bronchodilators
- Own PEF meter and if appropriate self management plan or written instructions for parents
- GP follow up arranged within 1 week
- Follow up appointment in clinic within 4 weeks

Adapted from poster designed by Business Design Group

In association with the General Practitioner in Asthma Group, the British Association of Accident and Emergency Medicine, the British Paediatric Respiratory Society and the Royal College of Paediatrics and Child Health

Figure 5.2 *(Continued)*.

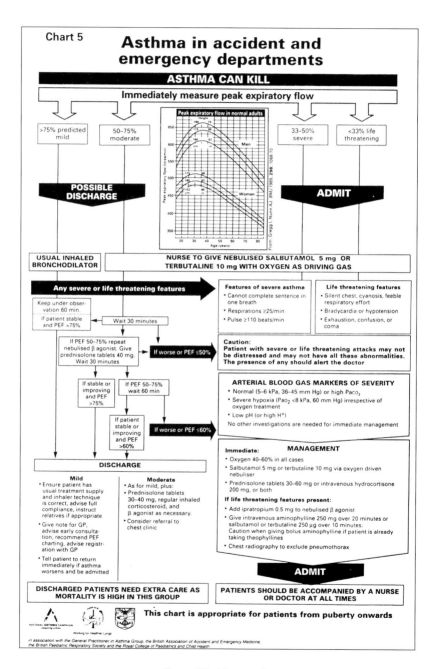

Chart 5 — Asthma in accident and emergency departments

ASTHMA CAN KILL

Immediately measure peak expiratory flow

| >75% predicted mild | 50–75% moderate | | 33–50% severe | <33% life threatening |

POSSIBLE DISCHARGE — **ADMIT**

Peak expiratory flow in normal adults — From Gregg I, Nunn AJ. BMJ 1989; 298: 1068–70

USUAL INHALED BRONCHODILATOR — **NURSE TO GIVE NEBULISED SALBUTAMOL 5 mg OR TERBUTALINE 10 mg WITH OXYGEN AS DRIVING GAS**

Any severe or life threatening features

Keep under observation 60 min.

If patient stable and PEF >75% — Wait 30 minutes

If PEF 50–75% repeat nebulised β agonist. Give prednisolone tablets 40 mg. Wait 30 minutes — **If worse or PEF ≤50%**

If stable or improving and PEF >75% — If PEF 50–75% wait 60 min

If patient stable or improving and PEF >60% — **If worse or PEF ≤60%**

DISCHARGE

Features of severe asthma
- Cannot complete sentence in one breath
- Respirations ≥25/min
- Pulse ≥110 beats/min

Life threatening features
- Silent chest, cyanosis, feeble respiratory effort
- Bradycardia or hypotension
- Exhaustion, confusion, or coma

Caution:
Patient with severe or life threatening attacks may not be distressed and may not have all these abnormalities. The presence of any should alert the doctor

ARTERIAL BLOOD GAS MARKERS OF SEVERITY
- Normal (5–6 kPa, 36–45 mm Hg) or high $Paco_2$
- Severe hypoxia (Pao_2 <8 kPa, 60 mm Hg) irrespective of oxygen treatment
- Low pH (or high H^+)
No other investigations are needed for immediate management

MANAGEMENT

Immediate:
- Oxygen 40–60% in all cases
- Salbutamol 5 mg or terbutaline 10 mg via oxygen driven nebuliser
- Prednisolone tablets 30–60 mg or intravenous hydrocortisone 200 mg, or both

If life threatening features present:
- Add ipratropium 0.5 mg to nebulised β agonist
- Give intravenous aminophylline 250 mg over 20 minutes or salbutamol or terbutaline 250 μg over 10 minutes. Caution when giving bolus aminophylline if patient is already taking theophyllines
- Chest radiography to exclude pneumothorax

Mild
- Ensure patient has usual treatment supply and inhaler technique is correct, advise full compliance, instruct relatives if appropriate
- Give note for GP, advise early consultation, recommend PEF charting, advise registration with GP
- Tell patient to return immediately if asthma worsens and be admitted

Moderate
- As for mild, plus:
- Prednisolone tablets 30–40 mg, regular inhaled corticosteroid, and β agonist as necessary.
- Consider referral to chest clinic

ADMIT

DISCHARGED PATIENTS NEED EXTRA CARE AS MORTALITY IS HIGH IN THIS GROUP — **PATIENTS SHOULD BE ACCOMPANIED BY A NURSE OR DOCTOR AT ALL TIMES**

NATIONAL ASTHMA CAMPAIGN — Working for Healthier Lungs

This chart is appropriate for patients from puberty onwards

In association with the General Practitioner in Asthma Group, the British Association of Accident and Emergency Medicine, the British Paediatric Respiratory Society and the Royal College of Paediatrics and Child Health

Figure 5.2 (Continued).

Chart 7

Acute episodes or exacerbations of asthma in young children in a community/primary care setting

Features of mild/moderate episode

β_2 agonist therapy: up to 10 puffs by metered dose inhaler + spacer (± face mask) at one puff every 15–30 seconds or by nebuliser 3–4 hourly

Responds favourably:

- respiratory rate reduced
- reduced use of accessory muscles
- improved "behaviour" pattern

Repeat every 3–4 hours
Consider doubling dose of inhaled steroids*

If still required 3–4 hourly after 12+ hours,** start a short course of prednisolone for 1–3 days
- <1 year 1–2 mg/kg/day
- 1–5 years 20 mg/day

Unresponsive or relapse within 3–4 hours

Increase frequency of β_2 agonist; give it as frequently as needed, while seeking further help; start oral prednisolone and move to Chart 8

Notes

* It is common practice to advise doubling of inhaled steroids early in the course of an attack, although there is no evidence for efficacy in young children.

** If there is experience of previous troublesome episodes in a particular child, a short course of prednisolone may be started earlier in an attack than indicated here. The efficacy of prednisolone in the first year of life is poor.

NATIONAL **ASTHMA** CAMPAIGN

Working for Healthier Lungs

In association with the General Practitioner in Asthma Group, the British Association of Accident and Emergency Medicine, the British Paediatric Respiratory Society and the Royal College of Paediatrics and Child Health

Figure 5.2 *(Continued).*

Chart 8

Acute severe asthma in children under 5 years of age

Recognition of acute severe asthma

Remember: • in preschool children there are other important causes of breathlessness and wheeze
• if you think a child has severe asthma, give β agonist at once

- Too breathless to talk
- Too breathless to feed
- Respirations > 50 breaths/min
- Pulse > 140 beats/min
- Use of accessory muscles of breathing

No other investigations are needed for immediate management; blood gas estimations are rarely helpful in deciding initial management in children

Life threatening features

- Cyanosis, silent chest, or poor respiratory effort
- Fatigue or exhaustion
- Agitation or reduced level of consciousness

Caution:
Children with severe attacks may not appear distressed; assessment in the very young may be difficult. The presence of any of these features should alert the doctor.

Management of a severe asthma attack

1 Immediate treatment

- High flow oxygen via face mask
- Salbutamol 2.5–5 mg or terbutaline 5–10 mg via an oxygen driven nebuliser (half doses in children under 1) or similar doses by spacer device.
- Prednisolone < 1 year 1–2 mg/kg/day; 1–5 years 20 mg/day
- Pulse oximetry is helpful. Sao_2 <92% in air indicates the need for admission.

IF LIFE THREATENING FEATURES OR POOR BRONCHODILATOR RESPONSE:

- Give intravenous aminophylline 5 mg/kg over 20 minutes followed by maintenance infusion of 1 mg/kg/h; omit the loading dose if child already receiving oral theophyllines
- Give intravenous hydrocortisone 100 mg 6 hourly
- Add ipratropium 0.25 mg to nebulised β agonist (0.125 mg in very young children)

2 Subsequent management

IF THE PATIENT IS IMPROVING CONTINUE:

- Oxygen to maintain Sao_2 >92%
- Prednisolone daily
- Nebulised β agonist 1–4 hourly

IF PATIENT IS NOT IMPROVING AFTER 15–30 MINUTES

- Continue oxygen and steroids
- Give nebulised β agonist more frequently, up to every 30 minutes
- Add ipratropium to nebuliser and repeat 6 hourly until improvement starts
- Consider need for chest radiography

IF PATIENT IS STILL NOT IMPROVING GIVE:

- Aminophylline infusion after loading dose if not already given; monitor blood concentrations if continued for over 24 hours.

3 Monitoring treatment

- Oximetry: maintain Sao_2 >92% Note clinical features at appropriate intervals.

4 Transfer to the intensive care unit accompanied by a doctor prepared to intubate if:

- Worsening or persistent hypoxia or hypercapnia
- Exhaustion, feeble respirations, confusion or drowsiness
- Coma or respiratory arrest

5 When discharged from hospital patients should have:

- Been stable on discharge medication for 6–8 hours and have had inhaler technique checked and recorded
- Treatment with soluble steroid tablets for total of 1–3 days
- Self management plan or written instructions for parents
- GP or hospital follow up arranged, with direct readmission for any deterioration within 24 hours.

 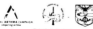

NATIONAL ASTHMA CAMPAIGN

Working for Healthier Lungs

In association with the General Practitioner in Asthma Group, the British Association of Accident and Emergency Medicine, the British Paediatric Respiratory Society and the Royal College of Paediatrics and Child Health

Adapted from poster designed by Business Design Group

Figure 5.2 *(Continued)*.

If available, beta-2 agonists should be given by a nebulizer, although multiple actuations of a pressurized metered dose inhaler, via a large volume spacer, can be equally effective[10]. If a spacer is used in this way, it is important that the patient inhales each puff separately, very soon after the inhaler has been actuated because of the very short half-life of respirable drug available for inspiration. Ipratropium bromide should be added in severe cases or in patients who show a poor response to beta-2 agonists. Nebulizer therapy should be withdrawn and replaced by an appropriate inhaler device as the patient improves. Occasionally intravenous beta-2 agonists may be beneficial.

In patients under the age of 50 and in older patients with no evidence of chronic obstructive pulmonary disease, high concentrations of oxygen (40–60%) should be given as this will not lead to carbon dioxide retention.

Inhalation devices

Delivery directly to the lungs, leading to rapid action and requiring a smaller dose with fewer side effects, makes inhalation the preferred route of administration for the majority of drugs used in the treatment of asthma. The range of inhaler devices (Figure 5.3; Table 5.2) available is testimony to there being no single device acceptable to all patients (see boxes).

It is difficult to use a pressurized metered dose inhaler device correctly and it requires careful instruction and reinforcement; there is no guarantee that patients will use them appropriately under the rigours of everyday life. Children under the age of 10 years, elderly patients, arthritic patients (Figure 5.4), and 30–50% of the normal population cannot use them appropriately. Even when patients use the best techniques, only 10–15% of the drug reaches the lung.

The ozone layer is being destroyed by chlorofluorocarbons (CFCs) in the stratosphere and by international agreement these are being phased out. CFCs are the propellants in the current pressurized metered dose inhalers. Although their contribution to the total source of CFCs was low in the past, pMDIs account for 96% of the current CFC usage in Europe.

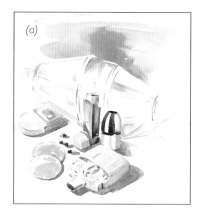
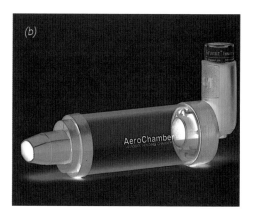

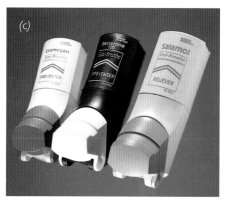

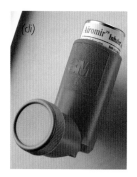
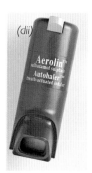
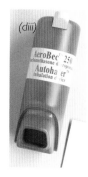

Figure 5.3 *Inhaler types. (a) Diskhaler, Rotahaler, pMDI and Volumatic spacer (Glaxo Wellcome); (b) Aerochamber (distributed by 3M Health Care Ltd; shown with Airomir pMDI); (c) Easi-breathe breath-actuated pMDIs (Glaxo Wellcome); (d)(i) Airomir, CFC-free pMDI; (ii) Aerolin Autohaler; (iii) Aerobec Autohaler (3M Health Care Ltd).*

Table 5.2 Inhaler devices

Device	Preventer	Reliever
pMDI + large volume spacer + mask	Beclomethasone Budesonide Fluticasone	Salbutamol Terbutaline Ipratropium
Large volume spacers:		
Volumatic	Beclomethasone Fluticasone	Salbutamol Salmeterol
Nebuhaler	Budesonide	Terbutaline
Fisonair	Sodium cromoglycate	
Aerochamber	All pMDIs	All pMDIs
pMDI	Not recommended alone in children	Not recommended alone in children
pMDI + large volume spacer	Beclomethasone Budesonide Fluticasone	Terbutaline Salbutamol Salmeterol Ipratropium
Breath-actuated dry powder devices:		
Turbohaler	Budesonide	Terbutaline
Rotahaler	Beclomethasone	Salbutamol
Diskhaler	Beclomethasone and Fluticasone	Salmeterol and Salbutamol
Spinhaler	Sodium cromoglycate*	
Accuhaler	Fluticasone	Salmeterol and Salbutamol
Aerohaler		Ipratropium bromide
Foradil inhaler		Eformoterol

Table 5.2 (Contd.)

Breath-actuated pMDIs:

Autohaler	Beclomethasone	Salbutamol, Ipratropium bromide Oxitropium, Fenoterol plus Ipratropium bromide
Easibreathe	Beclomethasone	Salbutamol

*Cromoglycate – not for children < 3 years of age
Abbreviation: pMDI = pressurized metered dose inhaler
(Adapted from the GPs in Asthma Group's Factsheet no.1, with permission from Dr Dermot Ryan, Chairman).

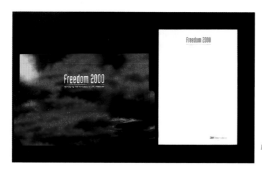

Figure 5.4 *A service in the UK, providing assistance for GPs in facilitating the transition from CFC to non-CFC inhalers. (Courtesy of 3M Health Care Ltd).*

Hydrofluoroalkane propellants (HFA-134a and HFA-127) have been developed to replace the CFCs and this has necessitated modifications to the design of the pressurized metered dose inhaler device with different delivery characteristics[31]. At the time of writing, the only non-CFC pressurized metered dose inhaler licensed in the United Kingdom is Airomir, containing salbutamol and utilizing HFA-134a as its propellant. The important message for our patients concerned about the change is that the HFAs are safer for the environment and as safe for humans as CFCs. The pressurized metered dose inhaler device is cheap and for

Inhaler devices for asthma: appropriate device types for different ages

Children aged 1–2 years
- pMDI with spacer + facemask
- nebulized therapy if above fails

Children aged >2 years
- pMDI with spacer
- pMDI with spacer + facemask
- If these methods fail, nebulized therapy

Children aged 5–8 years
- pMDI + spacer
- dry powder inhalers

Children >8 years and adults
- dry powder inhalers
- pMDI with spacer
- breath-actuated pMDI
- pMDI

Abbreviation: pMDI = pressurized metered dose inhaler

Problems with using a pressurized metered dose inhaler

- Correct inhalation technique
- Droplet size
- Deposition on oropharynx
- Lung deposition
- CFC propellants

many adult patients it is an effective form of treatment. Since beclomethasone dipropionate dissolves in HFA (and not CFC), the smaller particles produced have greater lung penetration and efficiency necessitating dosage adjustments. Initiatives such as 'Freedom 2000' (see Figure 5.4) aimed at simplifying the transition from prescribing of CFC to non-CFC inhalers should be useful to GPs during the transition period between CFC and HFA propellants.

A variety of inexpensive **spacer devices** have been developed for use with the pressurized metered dose inhalers. They have the advantage of reducing oropharyngeal and increasing lung disposition of the drug. The addition of a face mask allows spacer devices to be used in young children.

The **breath-actuated pressurized metered dose inhaler** is discharged at the start of inspiration by the patient and therefore requires less coordination. They are appropriate for patients unable to combine the act of actuation and inhalation effectively, i.e., those unable to use conventional pMDIs.

Dry powder devices were introduced to overcome the problems encountered in using the pressurized metered dose inhaler. They are all breath-actuated devices in which powdered drug is sucked into the lung during inspiration. Only the Turbohaler delivers pure drugs; the other devices have a mixture of the drug with a filler powder which facilitates inspiration. The devices vary in the inspiratory effort required, lung deposition achieved, dosing strength available and patient acceptability. The Turbohaler and Accuhaler, with their greater capacity for delivering multiple doses, have advantages over the Rotahaler and Diskhaler, although comparisons between the devices with regard to efficacy and acceptability are awaited.

The comparative monthly costs of administering different drugs through the various devices show considerable variation. While cost is a necessary consideration, it is just as important for patients to be treated with the most effective, appropriate combination (for them) of drug and device, even if this means selecting the most expensive.

Routine management of asthma with **nebulized** bronchodilators, sodium cromoglycate or budesonide, should only be considered as a last resort[10]. Nebulised therapy should be limited to those patients unable to use any of the other delivery systems because of age, incapacity or inability to coordinate the dual action of actuating and inhaling from the device.

There are a number of items that are useful for assisting or teaching patients how to use the inhaler devices and peak flow meters. The Haleraid (Figure 5.5) (Allen and Hanbury's), available for purchase from local pharmacies, is used with pressurized metered dose inhalers for those patients with joint problems in their hands. The device makes it easier to actuate the pressurized metered dose inhaler even if it is attached to a spacer. Vitalograph (Figure 5.6) manufacture a piece of equipment which is useful in assessing the different processes involved during inhalation of a drug: the speed of inspiration, the duration of inspiration and breath holding for an adequate time period. The Tri-Flo (Figure 5.7) is useful for teaching young children to inspire rather than blow out. The Windmill Trainer (Figure 5.8), which attaches to the low reading Mini-Wright Peak Flow Meter (Clement Clarke International Ltd) is useful for teaching children how to blow out when doing a peak flow measurement

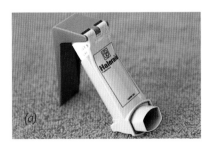

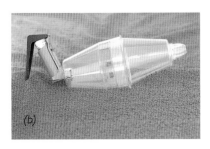

Figure 5.5 *The Haleraid (a) is useful for patients with arthritis and may be combined with a Volumatic (b).*

109

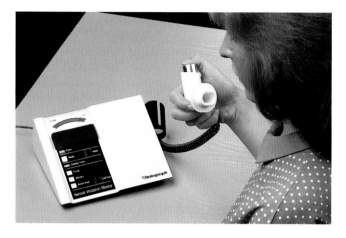

Figure 5.6 *Vitalograph manufacture a piece of equipment which is useful in assessing the different processes involved during inhalation of a drug; the speed of inspiration, the duration of inspiration and breath-holding for an adequate time period.*

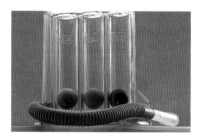

Figure 5.7 *The Tri-Flo is useful for teaching young children to inspire rather than blow out.*

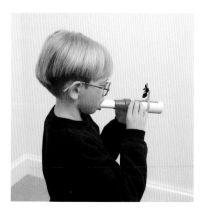

Figure 5.8 *The Windmill Trainer, which attaches to the low-reading Mini-Wright Peak Flow Meter (Clement Clarke International Ltd) is useful for teaching children how to blow out during a peak flow measurement.*

Each asthma clinic should have a whole range of devices in placebo form in order to check the patient's use of each device. The patient should be started on a device with which he or she is happy and can use effectively. The boxes summarize the delivery systems, the drugs and the appropriate ages for their use, and any problems that might be encountered (pages 105–107).

Rational approach to prescribing

Use of guidelines

To help our patients achieve optimum control of their asthma, we need to develop a rational and consistent approach to their management. By either following national guidelines, or adapting these to suit local conditions,[32] we may be able to achieve this goal.

A logical asthma consultation

An asthma consultation should be structured in such a way that logical treatment decisions may be taken to optimize the patient's asthma control. An example of a structured consultation was developed for use in a study to investigate the provision of care by hospital nurses for adults following an acute attack[33]. There are six steps to this process and they are shown in the box on page 112.

The structured consultation enables the health professional to determine logically whether the patient's current therapy needs to be adjusted up or down or continued as before. This is done first by establishing whether the patient has symptoms of asthma or unacceptably high peak flow variability. Then the peak flow variability is determined either from a diary card or by testing the peak flow or spirometry before and after a bronchodilator dose. Finally the patient's inhaler technique is tested in order to decide whether the device needs replacing with one more suitable for the person's ability. With all this information, a logical decision can be made whether or not to change the medication and a self-management plan can be agreed with the patient (see Figures 6.7a,b).

Advice before commencing inhaled steroids

Many patients are aware of the potential dangers of taking corticosteroids and may be apprehensive at the thought of starting long-term treatment even though it is with inhaled drugs. Patients need appropriate reassurance at an early stage as their need to use inhaled corticosteroids is likely to be long term[34]. Unless this issue is tackled properly, patient compliance with recommendations[17] is likely to be poor. The issues need to be discussed frankly and openly with each patient, noting any fears but emphasizing the relative safety of inhaled compared to oral corticosteroids. It is often useful to demonstrate symptomatic and functional improvement following the introduction of the inhaled steroids by means of diary cards and peak flow readings.

A six-step consultation in asthma[34]

1. Establish treatment step?
   - BTS Guidelines steps 0–5

2. Has patient any symptoms?
   - cough, wheeze, shortness of breath?
   - when do they occur?
   - how often do they occur?

3. Does patient use reliever medication?
   - once a day implies a need for preventer therapy

4. Peak flow variability?
   - % best or predicted
   - 15% implies poor asthma control

5. Inhaler technique?
   - score: preparation, inspiration, breath-holding.

6. Adjust therapy/change inhaler as appropriate and agree a self-management-plan?

Ongoing evaluation of provision of care

By incorporating a system of ongoing audit and evaluation of the care we provide, it may be possible to identify treatment approaches in need of revision. The latest review of the BTS Guidelines provide suggestions for outcome measures of asthma audit[10].

Chronic asthma: adults

In order to improve communication between health professionals, it seems sensible to develop and use universally accepted systems for scoring symptoms, inhaler technique, peak flow variability and treatment step. The latter could simply be the BTS treatment step with which many health professionals are already familiar.

The Tayside asthma stamp is now widely used in general practice for the purpose of standardizing symptom and peak flow scores (Figure 5.9).

The initial assessment should determine the maximum function the patient can achieve as a bench mark to aim at subsequently. In the case of peak flow, the patient's best ever readings should be used

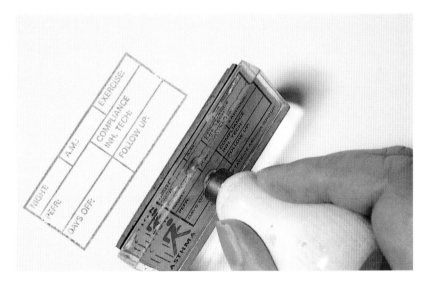

Figure 5.9 Dundee stamp. (Tayside Asthma Group. Reproduced with permission).

rather than the predicted ones, because of the lack of standardized national values applicable to the whole population. In addition, patients should be assessed on the same meter, preferably their own, because of the well recognized variability between meters. In some instances it may be necessary to give the patient a short course of oral steroids over two weeks in order to gauge the response (Figure 5.10).

The object of treatment is to reduce the symptoms and disability while maximizing respiratory function. Treatment should be in line with the recommendations in national guidelines[10–13].

It is currently recommended that patients with asthma should be started on the treatment step (BTS Guidelines) thought most likely to control their symptoms and then stepped down on the basis of their response to treatment[10]. Patients also need to understand that if their symptoms return then they need to increase the dose at an early stage in order to regain control.

The persistence of exercise-induced, nocturnal or morning symptoms in spite of improved overall control with prophylactic

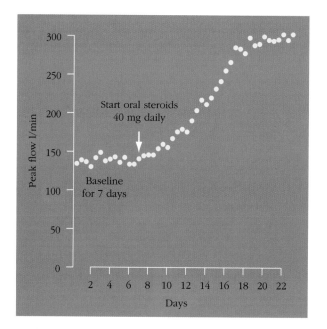

Figure 5.10 *Time for short course of oral steroids to take effect — 3/52 treatment showing slow increase in peak expiratory flow reading.*

medication may require appropriate adjunct therapy. Nocturnal, morning or twice daily salmeterol or formoterol may be effective in this situation; similarly oral theophyllines might be considered[25].

In those patients who present with persistent cough associated with asthma, there are strong theoretical reasons for considering the use of nedocromil sodium. This form of treatment may influence different components of the asthmatic inflammation — the eosinophil, the mast cell, the nerves and the epithelial cell — through a common mechanism involving the blockade of chloride channels. The drug is indicated for use in treating mild asthma, especially that associated with recurrent cough[36].

Asthma in children

Chronic

There are important differences in the patterns of symptoms and management of asthma in children and adults[10].

In most children with asthma, good long-term control of their symptoms can be achieved by using one or a combination of the following agents[10]:

■ beta-2 bronchodilators (short-acting for relief, long-acting for improved protection)
■ sodium cromoglycate
■ inhaled steroids
■ oral steroids.

As in adults, the inhaled route is always preferable: it offers more rapid onset of action, fewer side effects and requires a smaller dose than the oral route.

Other drugs are of limited value in children. Slow-release theophyllines (e.g. Slophylline 8–12 mg/kg twice daily) were used widely, but are now reserved for children with severe symptoms that are poorly controlled by inhaled corticosteroids. Although they are effective, side effects such as nausea, vomiting, sleep disturbance and poor concentration are common and severely limit their value; serum levels should be measured[37]. The inhaled anticholinergic bronchodilator ipratropium bromide (Atrovent) has a limited role in childhood asthma[18]. In some young infants with wheeze it is more effective than a short-acting beta-2 bronchodilator. Ipratropium is occasionally helpful in some older children with severe symptoms not controlled by inhaled steroids[38].

Antibiotics, cough medicines and decongestants are still widely used in asthma: they are of no proven value and they can produce significant side effects. Their use is also often associated with delay in introducing effective anti-asthma therapy. Antihistamines, such as loratadine (Clarityn) or cetirizine (Zirtek), can be helpful in the allergic rhinitis present in over a half of children with frequent or persistent asthma, but they do not improve the symptoms of asthma.

Selecting the drug regimen: The choice of treatment that is appropriate for an individual child is determined by the frequency and severity of their symptoms, by their age and, in some cases, by the factors that trigger their symptoms. There should be a logical step-wise progression of treatment, from the intermittent use of beta-2 bronchodilators for infrequent mild episodes, to high-dose inhaled steroids and oral prednisolone for the small minority of children with severe persistent asthma[1,10]. The point of entry (i.e. step two etc.) should be determined by the severity of symptoms at the time[10] and adjusted according to the child's response (see box).

Assessing the response to treatment in childhood asthma[1]

- Frequency of day-time and night-time cough and wheeze
- Limitation of exercise and other activities
- Days missed from school
- Frequency of need for relief treatment
- Frequency of acute attacks needing oral steroids or admission
- In older children with frequent symptoms, home peak expiratory flow readings.

To decide on appropriate treatment, it is often helpful to classify asthma by the pattern of symptoms in the child. In most cases, the asthma can be classified as:

- infrequent episodic asthma
- frequent episodic asthma
- persistent asthma.

Other patterns of symptoms include:

- exercise-induced asthma
- isolated nocturnal cough
- wheeze.

Infrequent episodic asthma

About three-quarters of asthmatic children have less than three or four episodes of wheeze and cough a year. Most episodes are triggered by a viral upper respiratory tract infection, especially in younger children. These children need no regular treatment. Episodes should be treated with an inhaled beta-2 bronchodilator, using an inhaler appropriate for the child's age. For severe attacks, nebulized bronchodilators and a short course of prednisolone (2–5 days) may be needed.

Frequent episodic asthma

About a fifth of asthmatic children have recurrent symptoms every 2–4 weeks. These children need regular inhaled preventative therapy and an inhaled beta-2 bronchodilator for relief. In the past, most guidelines recommended that prophylaxis should initially be with sodium cromoglycate given three to four times daily[1]. If there was no improvement within 4–6 weeks, it was suggested prophylaxis be changed to an inhaled steroid given twice-daily.

However, it is now evident that inhaled corticosteroids are the most effective preventative agents for children as well as adults with asthma. In conventional doses, their benefits far outweigh the small risk of local or systemic side effects. Most GPs and hospital doctors now use inhaled steroids as their first choice in children who need preventative therapy. This change in practice has been reflected by a steady increase in the number of prescriptions for inhaled steroids in children and a concomitant decline in the number of children prescribed sodium cromoglycate. The latest management guidelines reflect this change in practice[10]. The Pedersen group in Denmark have clearly demonstrated that children started on low-dose inhaled steroids at a early age have greater symptomatic and functional control on the lower dose of inhaled steroids than children in whom the decision to introduce inhaled steroids was delayed[23].

For most children, the inhaled steroid is started at 100–200 μg twice daily (using half this dose for the more potent fluticasone). In older children, and in those with more disturbing symptoms, it is reasonable to start with twice this dose. Once good symptom control has been achieved, it is often possible to step down the dose progressively towards half the initial level[23]. If there is an inadequate response, the dose of inhaled steroid may need to be doubled or even trebled. However, the risk of systemic side effects increases steeply once a daily dose of 800–1000 μg is exceeded; it is likely that there are different thresholds for unwanted effects in different children. An alternative approach is to add another drug, such as a long-acting beta-2 bronchodilator such as salmeterol, or a slow-release theophylline. Salmeterol is particularly effective in reducing troublesome nocturnal disturbance and exercise-induced symptoms in school-age children[38]. As it has no significant anti-inflammatory actions, it should be given only to children who are also taking inhaled corticosteroids.

In the unusual situation where frequent symptoms still persist, the child may need oral prednisolone to be added on a regular basis. A careful review of the diagnosis, inhaler technique, compliance, and the appearance of any avoidable trigger factors, such as the recent acquisition of a family pet, should always be performed before this serious step is taken in a child. All such children need regular monitoring of their asthma and growth in a specialist paediatric clinic. The dose of prednisolone should be carefully titrated against the clinical response so that the minimum can be used; in practice this is usually between 3–10 mg daily, depending on the size of the child. Although there is less impairment of growth with prednisolone given on alternate mornings, some patients can achieve adequate control only if they receive steroids each day.

Persistent asthma

Approximately 5% of asthmatic children have symptoms almost every day: if asked, they or their parents will say that they are rarely free of symptoms for longer than one or two days. All require regular prophylaxis with inhaled steroids and many will benefit from regular salmeterol. Long-standing symptoms may take weeks to improve: in some patients giving a course of oral prednisolone (1 mg/kg/day) for 10–14 days accelerates recovery. Some of these children need regular rather than intermittent beta-2 bronchodilator. Progression to continuous oral steroids may be necessary. Regular measurement of PEF is particularly helpful for assessing progress in this difficult group.

Other patterns of symptoms in childhood asthma

Some children have symptoms only on exertion, particularly in cold weather. Mild **exercise-induced** symptoms are often controlled by simply giving an inhaled beta-2 bronchodilator before exercise. For more severe exercise problems, a regular inhaled steroid or regular sodium cromoglycate, with an extra inhalation just before marked exertion such as physical exercise (PE) classes may be needed[38]. Salmeterol can be added to therapy for children who are on an inhaled steroid if their exercise-induced symptoms persist. Warm-up exercises before sports reduces exercise-induced bronchospasm.

The management of **the infant with recurrent wheeze and cough** is difficult. As previously discussed in Chapter 4, there are many possible causes of these symptoms. In some infants, the symptoms cause no distress and no treatment other than parental reassurance is needed. At the other end of the spectrum are infants who have recurrent episodes which result in repeated hospital admissions and frequent night-time disturbance for the child and family. If symptoms are causing distress to the child, rather than simply causing concern to the parents, then treatment should be given.

Decisions about drug therapy are more difficult in **infants** than in other age groups. Some drugs, such as sodium cromoglycate and oral bronchodilators, are of no proven value in infants[39]. Inhaled beta-2 agonists often produce no improvement in children <1 year old; indeed in some wheezy infants, nebulized bronchodilators can cause deterioration in lung function, although the mechanism for this paradoxical action remains unclear. The role of the long-acting bronchodilators in the very young child is not known. Ipratropium bromide improves lung function in some wheezy infants aged <18 months, but this is not necessarily paralleled by clinical improvement.

Inhaled steroids, given either by pressurized metered dose inhaler and large volume spacer in the same dose as in older children, or in the case of budesonide, by nebulizer, are effective in some infants with severe recurrent wheeze, cough and breathlessness.

Acute management

Recent national audits of the management of acute asthma attacks in general practice have revealed poor documentation of vital clinical parameters[40]. These observations may have been made; however, unless they are recorded, their significance is often missed. Many patients with a severe attack of asthma may not appear unduly distressed and it is only by recording the pulse rate, respiratory rate or peak flow readings that the true severity of the attack will be established. It is essential that such parameters are recorded when the patient is to be transferred from the primary to the secondary health care teams. The pulse rate is recognized as the most sensitive indicator of response to treatment. It shows improvement before any of the other parameters. Likewise, if the pulse rate rises it is an indicator that things are going wrong and treatment may need to be intensified or complications identified[41].

Patients with any features of acute severe or life-threatening asthma should be treated aggressively as indicated in Figure 5.2. Patients (a) with life-threatening asthma, (b) with acute severe asthma who fail to respond quickly to bronchodilators, (c) with an acute severe asthma attack showing significant nocturnal symptoms, seen in the evenings or weekend, (d) with poor comprehension of their illness, or (e) in adverse social circumstances, should be admitted at an earlier stage. Children with a PEF <40% of their predicted value, with an oxygen saturation of <92%, and who are becoming exhausted, need admission.

Assessment of severity in children: Except in infants, it is normally not difficult to diagnose acute asthma. Other causes of acute breathlessness, such as croup, acute epiglottitis or an inhaled foreign body, need to be considered.

It can be difficult to assess the severity of an acute attack in children.

Important points in the history include:

■ the duration of symptoms
■ what treatment has already been given
■ the course of previous attacks.

Wheeze and respiratory rate are unreliable indicators of severity: use of the accessory muscles (e.g. sternomastoids and alae nasi), chest retraction and pulse rate are better guides. Cyanosis indicates life-threatening asthma.

PEF is a helpful objective measure of severity and should be a routine part of the assessment but children below the age of five and those with severe dyspnoea usually cannot produce reliable readings. In A&E departments and in hospital wards, measurement of arterial oxygen saturation by pulse oximetry should be routine.

Treatment of children in hospital: As soon as the diagnosis has been made, the child should be given beta-2 adrenergic bronchodilator by nebulizer which should be driven by oxygen at a rate of 4–6 l/min. Depending on the response to treatment, this is repeated every $^1/_2$–2 hours until there is improvement and then the frequency of treatment may be progressively reduced. If nebulized treatment is unavailable, 5–10 puffs of a beta-2-adrenergic bronchodilator, given as one puff every 15–30 seconds through a spacer, is also effective.

Corticosteroids expedite recovery from acute asthma: oral prednisolone should be started in all children with the features of severe acute asthma. The normal loading dose is 1–2 mg/kg, with a maximum of 40 mg. This dose is repeated once daily for 2–5 days, depending on the rate of recovery. Teenagers, and particularly adolescent girls, may have exacerbations that are slow to resolve and they may require 7–10 days' therapy of prednisolone. There is no need to taper off the dose unless the child is on maintenance treatment with oral or high-dose inhaled steroids. Unless the child is vomiting, parenteral steroids offer no advantage over oral delivery. Antibiotics should be given only if there are clear signs of infection.

Intravenous aminophylline is now used infrequently and, although there is controversy about its value, it still has a role in the child who fails to respond adequately to intensive nebulized therapy. An intravenous loading dose (5 mg/kg) is given over 15 minutes (but omit if slow-release theophylline has been taken in the previous 12 hours), followed by a continuous infusion (1 mg/kg/h). The pulse and the cardiac rhythm should be monitored during infusion of the loading dose. Seizures, vomiting and cardiac arrhythmias may follow rapid infusion. Intravenous salbutamol is an alternative for children with life-threatening asthma that is not responding to maximal nebulized therapy, but should be used only in an ICU setting. Side effects include tachycardia and hypokalaemia. Unlike the situation with adults, there is no convincing evidence that adding nebulized ipratropium to maximal doses of nebulized beta-2 bronchodilators is beneficial in children.

Mechanical ventilation is rarely required in childhood asthma. In skilled hands, the prognosis is good. Children who require mechanical ventilation should be transferred to a paediatric ICU.

Before discharge, the child's maintenance treatment should be reviewed and altered if necessary. Inhaler technique should be checked. Follow-up by the GP or in the out-patient clinic should be arranged. Clear and prompt communication with the GP is essential (see Chapter 6) for children who require admission and for attendees to the A&E department with acute asthma.

Patients recovering from an acute asthma attack need careful monitoring until the clinical situation is stabilized. Therefore effective communication across the community–hospital interface is essential when patients are ready for discharge to their homes. Local development of protocols for transferring care across the interface may be helpful, in particular plans for stepping the therapy down once the patient starts improving.

Use of oral steroids

Oral corticosteroids, usually in short courses of 40–60 mg/day (adults) and 1–2 mg/kg/day (children) (maximum 40 mg/day) for 1–2 weeks, have several uses in the management of asthma as shown in the box.

Adult patients with moderately severe obstructive airways disease may not show great reversibility to bronchodilators but following a

---

Use of oral corticosteroids in asthma

- In a severe asthma attack
- In diagnosis
- To gain control
- To determine maximum function
- To treat failing control (fall in peak flow <60% of best / predicted)
  - worsening of nocturnal / morning symptoms
  - need for increasing amount of bronchodilators
  - diary card shows progressive worsening of symptomatic and functional control
- Daily prophylactic medication

---

course of oral steroids there may be a significant improvement in function allowing the diagnosis of asthma to be made (Figure 5.10). At the initial assessment a short course of steroids may be used to gain control before the patient is stabilized on prophylactic medications and to allow the determination of the maximum function achievable as a target for long-term care.

Judicious use of oral steroids are life saving in the acute situation. There are a few patients who require a small alternate day dose of oral steroids for long-term management providing alternative treatment has been maximized.

Self-management plans

Simply providing the patient with general factual information about asthma may increase knowledge but does not seem to improve morbidity or self management. To be effective an education programme should be personalized to the patient; it should contain practical advice on recognizing and treating uncontrolled asthma, and may be initiated through individual or group support sessions[42]. It is essential that patients and families of children with asthma understand the action of their prophylactic medication, the need for regular use and how to alter the dose according to circumstances, e.g. increasing it at the onset of a cold. The role of bronchodilator therapy needs to be clearly understood and the need for medical assistance if a patient does not get a rapid or sustained response. Most of the self-management plans are drawn up between community health-care professionals and the patient, with modifications as appropriate. However, in the acute situation, prior to discharge from hospital, it may be necessary to revise the plan. In such circumstances it is important that this information is transmitted to the primary care team.

Asthma is a condition that fluctuates and remits over time, and, therefore, it is sensible to transfer some of the responsibility of care to the patients and their families themselves. One of the methods employed is to provide patients with personally tailored asthma self-management plans. Various 'off the shelf' plans are available in the UK (Figure 5.11).

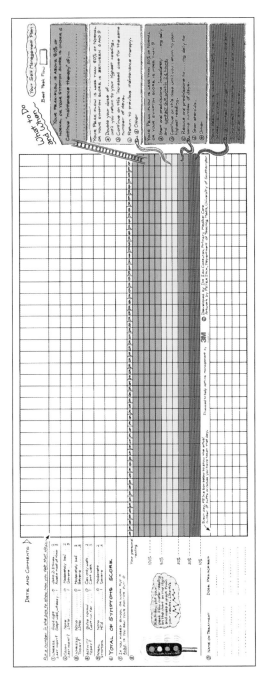

Figure 5.11 *Charlton self-management plan*[46,48]*. (Reproduced by permission of 3M Pharmaceuticals.)*

Alternatively, health professionals may design their own plan for example by using a PEF chart with action lines drawn at various levels (Figure 5.12)[43].

All of these plans incorporate similar principles which enhance patients' and their families' ability to recognize the signs of uncontrolled asthma and to take appropriate measures to prevent the development of attacks.

The use of written self-management plans (SMPs) became widespread following publication of an uncontrolled study[44], involving 36 consecutive outpatients. They were provided with 'peak flow action levels' which enabled them to double their inhaled corticosteroids or initiate a short course of oral corticosteroids if their peak flows dropped below 70% and 50% of best or predicted levels respectively. There was a substantial improvement in both subjective and objective measurements of asthma severity, with a significant reduction in nights woken, days lost from work and requirement for oral corticosteroids, and a significant increase in baseline lung function. This study indicated that routine measurement of PEF in association with a written self-management plan appears to be effective in reducing symptoms of asthma and improving lung function, and paved the way for the development and enhancement of the idea. Since then there have been a number of studies confirming the benefits of providing patients with a SMP[45-59].

Although there are many self-management plans from which to choose, we have elected to describe the National Asthma Campaign (NAC) plans for adults in detail in order to demonstrate their use. The adult plan (Figure 5.13) is divided into four zones and helps the patient to confirm that their asthma is well controlled (Zone 1) and to identify three levels of uncontrolled asthma (Zones 2, 3 and 4). Similar plans are available for children.

In addition, each zone is accompanied by instructions to take appropriate measures. Zone 2 is intended for use when the peak flow drops by 20% or where the patient requires more relief medication or has developed symptoms.

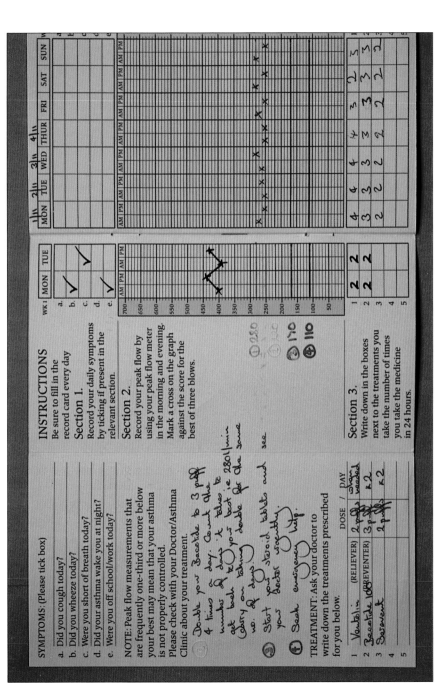

Figure 5.12 *Hayward–Levy lines on charts*[43].

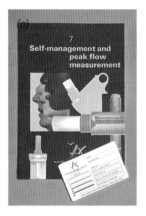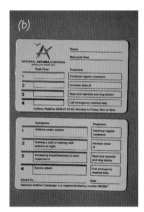

Figure 5.13 *NAC Credit Card.*

Appropriate follow-up

Most patients with chronic asthma may be assessed and managed by the primary care team, preferably in a well-resourced asthma clinic run by a trained asthma nurse. In some circumstances advice may be sought from the local respiratory physician or a patient may require hospital admission in an acute severe attack. Under these circumstances good communication between the primary and secondary care team is essential.

The frequency with which patients are followed in primary care or the hospital sector depends on the nature of their asthma. Studies have shown that following the initial assessment several visits may be required in order to stabilize the patient's asthma and develop management plans. Once this stage is passed then the frequency of follow-up becomes much less. Patients with mild asthma may only need to be seen yearly, or even on an as-required basis. Each clinic needs to have an appropriate recall system to ensure that patients are appropriately seen and that identifying and contacting defaulters is systematic.

The aims of good management in asthma must be to ensure morbidity is reduced to the minimum and that the patient achieves maximum functional ability. Each individual is different and must be approached on a one-to-one basis. Ultimately, the patient should be empowered to manage their own asthma under the direction of the primary care team. The principles of management outlined in this chapter should help to achieve these objectives.

References

1 British Thoracic Society *et al.* Guidelines for the management of asthma: a summary. *BMJ* 1993; **306**: 776–82.

2 Anonymous. Guidelines on the management of asthma. Statement by the British Thoracic Society, the British Paediatric Association, the Research Unit of the Royal College of Physicians of London, the King's Fund centre, the National Asthma Campaign, the Royal College of General Practitioners, the General Practitioners in Asthma Group, the British Association of Accident and Emergency Medicine, and the British Paediatric Respiratory Group [published errata appear in *Thorax* 1994; **49**: 96 and 1994; **49**: 386]. *Thorax* 1993; **48**: S1–24.

3 McCowan C *et al.* The facilitator effect: results from a 4 year follow up of children with asthma. *Br J Gen Pract* 1997; **47**: 156–60.

4 Murray AD, Morrison BJ. Effect of cigarette smoke from the mother on bronchial responsiveness and severity of symptoms in children with asthma. *J Allergy Clin Immunol* 1986; **75**: 575.

5 Couriel JM. Passive smoking and the health of children. *Thorax* 1994; **49**: 731–4.

6 Silverman M. Out of the mouths of babes and sucklings: lessons from early childhood asthma. *Thorax* 1993; **48**: 1200–4.

7 Millar K. Sensitivity to tartrazine. *BMJ* 1982; **285**: 1597.

8 Ayres JG, Clark TJH. Alcoholic drinks and asthma: a survey. *Br J Dis Chest* 1983; **77**: 370.

9 Widal MF, Abrami P, Lermoyez J. Anaphylaxie et idiosyncrasie. *Presse Med* 1922; **30**: 189–94.

10 British Thoracic Society, The National Asthma Campaign, The Royal college of Physicians of London, The General Practitioner's in Asthma Group, The British Association of Accident and Emergency Medicine, The British Paediatric Respiratory Society. British Guidelines on Asthma Management: 1995 Review and position statement. *Thorax* 1997; **52** (Suppl.): S1–21.

11 Scheffer A. Global strategy for asthma management and prevention *NHLBI/WHO Workshop Report.* 1995; 95-3659: 1–176.

12 Anonymous. International consensus report on diagnosis and treatment of asthma. National Heart, Lung and Blood Institute, National Institutes of Health. Bethesda, Maryland 20892. Publication no. 92-3091, March 1992. *Eur Resp J* 1993; **5**: 601–41.

13 Spelman R. Guidelines for the diagnosis and management of asthma in general practice. *Irish Coll Gen Pract* 1996;1–34.

14 Sheffer AL, Taggart VS. The national asthma education program. Expert panel report. Guidelines for the diagnosis and management of asthma. National Heart, Lung and Blood Institute. *Med Care* 1993; **31**: MS20-8.

15 Couttes JAP, Gibson NA, Paton NY. Measuring compliance with inhaled medication in asthma. *Arch Dis Child* 1992; **67**: 332–3.

16 Price DB. Inhaled steroid prescribing over seven years in a general practice and its implications. *Eur Resp J* 1995; 19 (Suppl.): 463s.

17 Barnes PJ, Pedersen S. Efficacy and safety of inhaled corticosteroids in asthma. Report of a workshop held in Eze, France, October 1992. *Am Rev Resp Dis* 1993; **148**: S1–26.

18 Pedersen S. Clinical pharmacology and therapeutics. In: Silverman M, ed. *Childhood asthma and other wheezing disorders*. London: Chapman & Hall, 1995.

19 Price JF. The role of inhaled fluticasone propionate, efficacy and safety. *Eur Resp Rev* 1996; **6**: 204–7.

20 Russell G. Inhaled corticosteroid therapy in children: an assessment of the potential for side effects. *Thorax* 1994; **49**: 1185–8.

21 Agertoft L, Pedersen S. Importance of the inhalation device on the effect of budesonide. *Arch Dis Child* 1994; **69**: 130–3.

22 Borgstrom L, Derom E, Stahl E, Wahlin-Boll E, Pauwels R. The inhalation device influences lung deposition and bronchodilating effect of terbutaline. *Am J Resp Crit Care Med* 1996; **153**: 1636–40.

23 Agertoft L, Pedersen S. Effects of long term management with an inhaled steroid on growth and pulmonary function in asthmatic children. *Resp Med* 1994; **88**: 373–81.

24 Holgate ST, Bradding P, Sampson AP. Leucotriene antagonists and synthesis inhibitors: New directions in asthma therapy. *J All Clin Immunol* 1996; **98**: 1–13.

25 Greening AP, Ind PW, Northfield M, Shaw G. Added salmeterol versus higher dose corticosteroids in asthma patients with symptoms on existing inhaled corticosteroids. *Lancet* 1994; **344**: 219–24.

26 O'Driscoll BR *et al.* Nebulised salbutamol with and without ipratropium bromide in acute airflow obstruction. *Lancet* 1989; **1**: 1418–20.

27 Sullivan TJ. Anti-Inflammatory effects of low dose oral theophylline in atopic asthma. *Lancet* 1994; **343**: 1006–8.

28 Office of Population Censuses and Surveys. Morbidity statistics from general practice 1991/92 (MSGP4). *OPCS Monitor* 1994; MB5 **94/1**: 1–12.

29 Central Health Monitoring Unit. *Asthma. An epidemiological overview.* London: HMSO, 1995; pp. 1–61.

30 British Thoracic Society. Guidelines for management of asthma in adults: II – acute severe asthma. *BMJ* 1990; **301**: 797–800.

31 Hayman G. Ozone depletion and CFCs in asthma inhalers. *Asthma Care Today* 1995; **3**: 32–4.

32 Scottish Intercollegiate Guidelines Network. Hospital in-patient management of acute asthma attacks. 1996; **6**: 1–29.

33 Levy M, Allen J, Doherty C, Winter R. The asthma consultation: A six step guide. In: *Anonymous distance learning pack.* The NATC/RCGP Diploma. Stratford-upon-Avon: National Asthma Training Centre, 1995.

34 Merkus PJ, van Essen-Zandvliet EE, Duiverman EJ, Van Houwelingen HC, Kerrebijn KF, Quanjer PH. Long-term effect of inhaled corticosteroids on growth rate in adolescents with asthma. *Pediatrics* 1993; **6**: 1121–6.

35 Loftus BG, Price JF. Treatment of preschool children with slow release theophylline. *Arch Dis Child* 1995; **60**: 770–2.

36 Report on the Working Groups for the Canadaian Asthma Concensus Conference. *Can Resp J* 1996; **13** (Suppl. B): 19B–20B.

37 Couriel JM. Management of asthma. *Curr Paed* 1991; **1**: 30–5.

38 Green CP, Price JF. Prevention of exercise induced asthma by inhaled salmeterol. *Arch Dis Child* 1992; **67**: 1014–17.

39 Silverman MS, Wilson NM. Wheezing disorders in infancy. In: Silverman M, ed. *Childhood asthma and other wheezing disorders.* London: Chapman & Hall, 1995.

40 Neville RG, Clark RC, Hoskins G, Smith B. National asthma attack audit 1991–2. General Practitioners in Asthma Group [see comments]. *BMJ* 1993; 306: 559–62.

41 Mathur R, Clark RA, Dhillon DP, Winton JH, Lipworth BJ. Re-audit of acute asthma admissions using a severity marker stamp and determinants of an outcome measure. *Scott Med J* 1997 **42**: 49–52.

42 Partridge MR. Delivering optimal care to the person with asthma: what are the key components and what do we mean by patient education?. [Review]. *Eur Resp J* 1995; **8**: 298–305.

43 Hayward SA, Levy M. Patient self management of asthma [letter]. *Br J Gen Pract* 1990; **40**: 166.

44 Beasley R, Cushley M, Holgate ST. A self management plan in the treatment of adult asthma. *Thorax* 1989; **44**: 200–4.

45 Bailey WC, Richards JM Jr, Brooks CM, Soong SJ, Windsor RA, Manzella BA. A randomized trial to improve self-management practices of adults with asthma. *Arch Intern Med* 1990; **150**: 1664–8.

46 Charlton I, Charlton G. New perspectives in asthma self-management. *Practitioner* 1990; **234**: 30–2.

47 Brewis RA. Patient education, self-management plans and peak flow measurement. [Review]. *Resp Med* 1991; **85**: 457–62.

48 Charlton I. Self-management plans for asthma control. *Nursing Times* 1991; 87: 52.

49 Muhlhauser I, Richter B, Kraut D, Weske G, Worth H, Berger M. Evaluation of a structured treatment and teaching programme on asthma. *J Int Med* 1991; **230**: 157–64.

50 Wilson SR, Scamagas P, German DF *et al.* A controlled trial of two forms of self-management education for adults with asthma. *Am J Med* 1993; **94**: 564–76.

51 Anon. Effectiveness of routine self monitoring of peak flow in patients with asthma. Grampian asthma study of integrated care (GRASSIC). *BMJ* 1994; **308**: 564–7.

52 Charlton I, Antoniou AG, Atkinson J *et al.* Asthma at the interface: bridging the gap between general practice and a district general hospital. *Arch Dis Child* 1994; **70**: 313–18.

53 D'Souza W, Crane J, Burgess C *et al.* Community-based asthma care: trial of a "credit card" asthma self-management plan. *Eur Resp J* 1994; **7**: 1260–5.

54 Partridge MR. Asthma: guided self management. *BMJ* 1994; **308**: 547–8.

55 Allen RM, Jones MP, Oldenberg B. Randomised trial of an asthma self-management programme for adults. *Thorax* 1995; **50**: 731-8.

56 Ignacio-Garcia JM, Gonzalez-Santos P. Asthma self-management education program by home monitoring of peak expiratory flow. *Am J Resp Crit Care Med* 1995; **151**: 353–9.

57 Levy ML, Robb M, Allen J, Doherty C, Bland M, Winter RJD. Guided self-management reduces morbidity, time off work and consultations for uncontrolled asthma in adults. *Eur Resp J* 1995 (Suppl.); **19**: 318s.

58 Hayward SA, Jordan M, Golden G, Levy M. A randomised controlled evaluation of asthma self management in general practice. *Asthma Gen Pract* 1996; **4**: 11–13.

59 Lahdensuo A, Haahtela T, Herrala J *et al.* Randomised comparison of guided self management and traditional treatment of asthma over one year. *BMJ* 1996; **312**: 748–52.

Chapter 6

Towards a seamless interface

The provision of asthma care in the UK has changed dramatically over the last decade. There have been several factors that have stimulated this change. For example, in 1982, the British Thoracic Association (BTA), in its study on 90 asthma deaths in adults, highlighted major deficiencies in the management of acute asthma[1]. In over 80% of cases, there was a failure of the doctors, the patients and their relatives to recognize the severity of the attack. In addition, in many cases, once the diagnosis had been made, the treatment given was inadequate. Most of the deaths were regarded as potentially avoidable. Inadequate training in asthma management and poor organization of asthma care in the early 1980s were thought to be explanations for these errors. Organized care for people with asthma, such as dedicated clinics, took place only in specialist respiratory units in hospitals and in very few, innovative primary care centres. At that time few GPs provided any organized care for patients with chronic diseases such as diabetes, hypertension or asthma[2]. It is now recognized that advice by different health professionals must be consistent and complementary if we are to enhance effectively patients' knowledge of their illness. There needs to be consistent management and advice across the hospital–community interface.

In this chapter, we discuss the asthmatic patient's use of health services and ways to encourage their appropriate use. We will consider aspects of organization of asthma care as well as communication and referral across the community and hospital interfaces of asthma care.

133

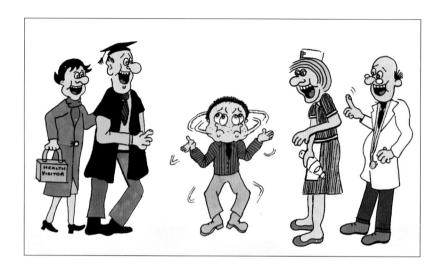

The BTA study[1] was a major landmark in asthma management and one of the factors that led to the development of organized primary care for asthmatic people. Robert Pearson, a GP, and Greta Barnes MBE, a practice nurse, developed their innovative asthma clinic[3] which had its roots in their experience in nurse-run hypertension clinics[4]. Mrs Barnes subsequently founded the National Asthma and Respiratory Training Centre (NARTC) in Stratford-upon-Avon (now Warwick) which currently provides diploma level asthma training for nurses, as well as training in other aspects of respiratory care for nurses and doctors.

The most important influence on the management of asthma in children in the 1980s was a study in Tyneside[5], which highlighted the underdiagnosis and undertreatment of asthma. This study established the prevalence of childhood asthma at about 11%, raised awareness of the disruption that undiagnosed asthma caused and confirmed the importance of using the diagnostic label as previously noted by Anderson *et al.*[6]. Furthermore, this study stimulated a number of primary care studies[7–12], which, in turn, stimulated considerable further development of primary care for people with asthma.

Other major initiatives in improving asthma management in the UK in the last ten years include the founding of the GPs in Asthma Group (GPIAG)[13], the development of protocols for asthma management by the Royal College of GPs[14] and British (known as the BTS) guidelines[15–18]. The GPIAG provides a forum for interested GPs to initiate, coordinate and share results of asthma audit and research, and develop ideas for improved care. The guidelines provide a framework for care to be used in their original format or alternatively to be adapted locally for implementation.

The advent of the NARTC and the introduction of payment, in the UK in 1990, for general practices to provide organized care in clinics led to an expansion in the numbers of nurse-run asthma clinics. A growing number of studies have demonstrated that organized care reduces patient morbidity and workload of GPs[3,19–24].

As a result of changes in the structure of the NHS there is a tendency to establish outreach clinical services in a primary healthcare setting and emphasis on better communication between the GP and the hospital specialist. In children, an increasing number of district paediatric units now run asthma clinics. In the last five years the appointment of specialist asthma nurses in the hospital and more recently in the community, has led to improved education and advice for the families of children with asthma. In Glasgow and Central Scotland, an audit showed 20–25% childhood asthma admissions were readmissions, a figure confirmed from Tayside. The introduction of a paediatric/respiratory liaison nurse providing education, facilitating discharge and providing support in the community, has reduced the readmission rate from 25% to 8%[25]. However, hospital admissions for acute asthma, especially in children, continue to increase. Whether this reflects increased reluctance by GPs to treat acute asthma in the community, or increased awareness of the consequences of acute asthma, or a combination of both, is not known. The use of A&E departments by patients with acute asthma is still high, suggesting that patients' use of care for asthma in the primary healthcare setting is still far from perfect. In the ideal world, few patients with asthma would need to attend their local hospital department.

Some asthmatic patients with atypical or severe symptoms do need to be referred for specialist advice. However, in most cases, the GP could meet all the clinical needs of their asthmatic patients, with a degree of flexibility, continuity and availability of care that can rarely be matched in hospital. In many practices, this ideal of community-based, patient-centred care is a reality, but in others, the lack of such a level of care leads to asthma that is poorly controlled, and results in repeated visits to the A&E department or admissions to hospital and inappropriate referrals to out-patient clinics.

There are many possible explanations for these poor levels of asthma control. Standards of care and levels of nurse training differ[26] and the quality of care provided by doctors varies considerably[27–34]. As with any chronic disorder, poor patient compliance and adherence to treatment is common and contributes to inadequate control of symptoms. There are complex factors (see box) which may explain this sort of behaviour[35].

A substantial proportion of patients fail to attend for follow-up appointments after hospital admission for acute asthma[36]. Patients who

Factors in non-adherence to medical advice.

- Lack of understanding
- Unrealistic or frustrated expectations
- Depression
- Denial of illness
- Peer pressure
- Shame/embarrassment
- Low socioeconomic status
- Anger
- Literacy
- Isolation

need to be seen regularly but who fail to attend require special attention. In one study poor follow-up attendance was associated with low socioeconomic status, illiteracy, ethnicity and occupational asthma[37]. A community study of 20–45-year-old patients, with moderately severe asthma symptoms and significant morbidity, who had failed to contact health professionals for advice, suggested that a major deterrent to them seeking advice was that they anticipated disapproval of their lifestyle, for example their smoking habits[38].

Patient awareness and empowerment has been enhanced by the efforts of the National Asthma Campaign (NAC); a registered UK charity, which is dedicated to increasing knowledge and awareness and improvement of asthma care, through education of patients as well as health professionals, and by raising funds for asthma research. The use of self-management plans is one way of empowering patients that has aroused considerable interest worldwide over the last decade (see Chapter 5).

Current organization of asthma care in the UK

At present the standard of asthma care varies considerably throughout the UK. There has been a considerable shift from secondary to primary care without an increase in adequate resources or enhanced training of healthcare personnel. Like other chronic disease management, asthma care varies according to the experience and expertise of those providing it. In hospital, asthmatic patients are treated in A&E departments as well as in general medical, general paediatric or specialist respiratory units. In general practice, patients are treated by doctors or nurses who have different levels of expertise and experience in asthma management.

Effective management depends on the relationship between the patient, their GP and other members of the primary care team, including practice nurses, health visitors and receptionists. Most patients with asthma receive all their care within the community.

However, patient contact with the primary care team differs from practice to practice. In a well-established, nurse-run asthma clinic, initial patient contact may be made directly with the nurse who will either deal with the problem or arrange for the GP to do so. In either event, patients should not be made to feel that they have failed if things go wrong and they suffer attacks, rather that the team is there to support and encourage them. Receptionists, who are often the first point of contact, play a key role in assisting patients to obtain help when their asthma is out of control.

Acute episodes of asthma

Patients' use of services follows at least three patterns for acute asthma episodes:

■ Patients seek help from their GPs[28] who sometimes refer them to hospital

■ they go directly to an A&E department or

■ some patients with severe or brittle asthma have the facility to access specialist care directly by self-admission.

In a national acute asthma audit[28], over 1800 attacks were managed exclusively in general practice. There were no significant differences in management between practices with a stated interest in asthma (GPIAG members) and those recruited via national adverts. However, three other studies of acute asthma episodes found that 66% (859/1292)[39], 80% (186/233)[40] and 73% (155/211)[36] of the patients respectively referred themselves directly to the A&E departments without contacting their GPs. A significant proportion of patients in these three studies were admitted to hospital and many of them reattended the A&E departments, 39% within three months[39], 17% within two months[40], and 35% within 13 months[40], respectively. It is not clear whether this group of patients who attend A&E departments is typical of the more severe asthmatics, or whether they have a poor awareness or availability of access to their GPs. In one audit in Manchester, parents were asked why they had brought their children to A&E department rather than consult their GP.

In reply the parents said that:

■ the GP would simply have referred them to hospital
■ they could not get to see their doctor urgently
■ their GP did not know about asthma.

While results of a local audit like this may not reflect the opinions of the population, they do provide us with an explanation for some patients' self-management behaviour. Repeated reattendance at the A&E departments indicates poor asthma control. Referral of recurrent attendees by these departments, either to their GP or to a specialist hospital clinic, may result in improved asthma management. In this way we may improve the care of these patients, reduce the risk of death resulting from attacks (by preventing the attacks through enhanced treatment) and reduce wasteful misuse of scarce resources — most of these patients should be treated in primary care.

The standard of care for acute episodes varies considerably and there is evidence that this could be improved. The GPIAG study[28] showed that despite a stated interest in asthma, over 50% of the attacks were not managed according to the published national guidelines[16,17], although there was widespread acceptance of these by the membership of the group[41]. Studies on asthma deaths continue to show marked deficiencies in care delivered by hospitals[32,42,43] and GPs[27], particularly in terms of measurement of lung function and use of appropriate anti-asthma medication. Bucknall *et al* showed that there were marked differences in the provision of acute care by adult physicians with a respiratory interest compared with generalists[33,34], although this had improved by the time the audit cycle was completed[31].

Improving acute care

Health districts may be able to improve acute asthma care by trying different approaches to organization of services.

Use of pro-forma asthma records

In our experience, non-adherence by health professionals to protocols and guidelines is a problem in the care of acute asthmatic patients. In addition, retrospective audit of the process and delivery of A&E department care is difficult, complicated by the individualistic way in which doctors record their clinical findings and treatment. This may be overcome by using pro-forma medical record flow sheets with check boxes, and advice on management. This approach may lead to improvement of care by guiding junior staff through the management of the patient and by providing a means of reliable audit of care. For example, Town *et al*[4] developed a standardized management protocol record sheet (Figure 6.1a and b) for the assessment and treatment of adults with acute asthma attending an emergency department in Wellington, New Zealand. This enabled recording of essential features of the history and examination findings and provided a flow diagram with guidelines for initial management that were based on spirometry recordings. Analysis of emergency department records during the three months before and one year after the introduction of the protocol showed that there were improvements in history-taking, increased use of serial measures of airflow obstruction and improved documentation of follow-up arrangements. The provision of management guidelines influenced the emphasis of management, including an increased use of corticosteroids intravenously and more frequent use of an additional dose of nebulized bronchodilator.

Specially designed record cards and sheets in general practice and in acute medical and paediatric hospital units may improve adherence to protocols and aid audit which has the aim of improving acute care. Figure 6.2 demonstrates an example of an asthma admission pro forma developed by the Brighton Paediatric Asthma Research Team. Although data has not yet been published, the paediatric senior house officers using this form seem to be quite happy with it. Figure 6.3 shows a patient-held record card for asthma in childhood designed by the Enfield Children's Asthma Coordinating Committee.

Various other examples of record sheets are shown in this chapter (Figures 6.4–6.6). An idea, which is to be piloted in London soon, is the use of a referral pro-forma sheet that would serve as a means of communication between health professionals as well as a prospective audit data collection sheet.

ASTHMA ASSESSMENT SHEET
(To be placed in the accident and emergency department (A&E card); copy with patient)

Name		Date	
Hospital number		Time of arrival	
Name of GP			

Asthma History

Usual Medication (dose and frequency)

Duration of current attack		Beta$_2$ agonist	
		Inhaled steroid	
Number of attacks in previous 12 months		Theophylline	
		Other	
Previous ICU admission	Yes (tick)		
	No		
Use of corticosteroids	Previous courses of prednisone		
	Maintenance prednisone	Predicted VC	
		Predicted FEV$_1$	

Progress Record

Data	Initial assessment	After 15 minutes	Final assessment
Time			
Pulse rate			
FEV$_1$ litres			
% predicted			
Treatment given			

Inhaler technique checked: Satis / Poor

Comments: _____

_____

_____

_____

Follow up arrangements: _____

_____

_____

Discharge medications:

_____
Casualty officer's name

Figure 6.1a *A&E department proforma for use by A&E department staff when recording information in the medical records.*[44]

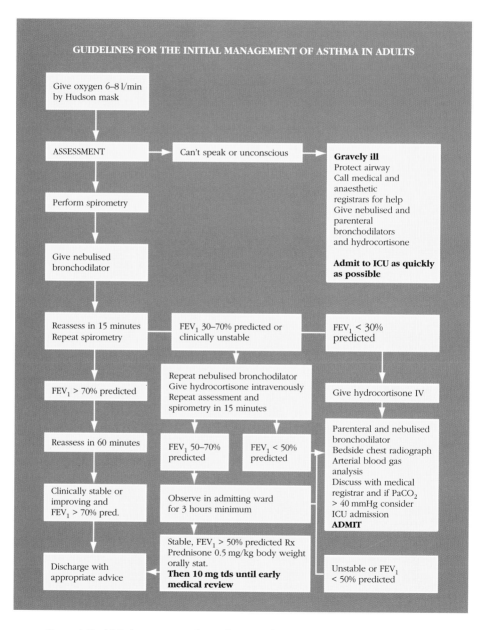

Figure 6.1b A&E department proforma for use by A&E department staff when recording information in the medical records.[44]

The form is first completed by the GP who keeps a copy. The document then goes with the patient to hospital where the A&E or relevant on-call team completes the next section and the process continues until the patient is discharged with a copy of the complete form for the GP's records. Figure 6.4 is a similar example, whereby an acute asthma book is kept. This was developed by Mary White, an asthma facilitator in Cornwall. The book is used for all patients admitted to hospital with an asthma attack. The data are recorded in the book and then a copy is sent to the GP who completes the section detailing the action taken at the follow-up visit to the practice. The form is not filed in the medical records until the patient has been seen and therefore serves as a reminder for the practice staff to ensure that efforts are made to contact non-attendees[45].

Ensuring and using appropriate training for staff

GPs commonly complain that patients referred acutely to hospital are seen by inexperienced staff. When a GP requires a second opinion, ideally a senior hospital doctor (one with training in asthma care) should see the patient, possibly as a joint consultation with the junior on call. This approach was beneficial at the Brighton hospital[46] when the on-call senior house officer (SHO) was replaced by an experienced registrar in casualty. In the four-month study period the registrar doubled the proportion of children sent home compared with that of the SHOs. This study was followed by an SHO training programme and the development of a home treatment package. This resulted in a substantial increase, over 12 months, in the proportion of children with acute asthma deemed fit to be sent home. Few of these were readmitted within one week of attendance and diary symptom score cards (for two weeks after discharge) indicated that children sent home without admission fared no worse at home than those admitted. Longer term studies of this nature may assist future planning for provision of care.

As so many patients refer themselves to the A&E department with uncontrolled asthma, it may be appropriate to provide training for all (or some) members of the nursing staff working in these departments.

ASTHMA ADMISSION SHEET (Front)

Child's details	Date of birth:	K no.:
Surname:	Date seen in casualty:	Time seen in casualty:
First name:	Referral Source:	Admitting SHO:
Address:	GP address:	Consultant: JT PS NE
		Religion:
Post code:	Post code:	Health visitor:
Telephone No.:	Telephone No.:	School:

Presenting history.

Duration of presenting symptoms
Cough for.........days   Shortness of breath for............days   Wheeze for........days   Cold for.........days.

Sent home from A+E (or equivalent) in previous 24hrs: ☐ Yes ☐ No

Asthma symptoms in previous 6 months

Night time cough:

☐ Less than twice a month

☐ 1-2 x per week

☐ More than 3 x per week

Wheeze on waking:

☐ Less than twice a month

☐ 1-2 x per week

☐ More than 3 x per week

Activity induced symptoms:

☐ Occasional

☐ Everytime

☐ Even after bronchodilator

Effect on quality of life, in parent/child's opinion:

☐ None

☐ Mild

☐ Moderate

☐ Severe

No. days off school/nursery: ☐   No. of GP consultations: ☐

Asthma history
Age asthma diagnosed (yrs):.........   Age first symptomatic (yrs):.......   Age first given oral steroids (yrs):.......

Number of previous asthma admissions:........   Bronchiolitis in infancy: ☐ Yes ☐ No

Ever admitted to ITU? ☐ Yes ☐ No   Ever ventilated? ☐ Yes ☐ No   Home nebuliser source: ☐ None ☐ Own ☐ Hospital ☐ GP ☐ Other

Triggers
☐ URTI   ☐ Cold air   ☐ Exercise   ☐ Emotion   ☐ House dust
☐ Pets   ☐ Feathers   ☐ Food   ☐ Smoking   ☐ Others...................

Birth history/Past medical history
Gestation (wks):...........   Birth weight (kgs):.........   IPPV for ....days   Oxygen for............days   Breast fed
for.........weeks

Allergy to medication: Social/family history:

Any other illnesses and consultant:

Immunisations:

Development:

Family/home history

Asthma:
☐ Mother
☐ Father
☐ Self
☐ Siblings

Eczema:
☐ Mother
☐ Father
☐ Self
☐ Siblings

Hayfever:
☐ Mother
☐ Father
☐ Self
☐ Siblings

Smoking:
☐ Mother
☐ Father
☐ Self
☐ Siblings

Pets:
☐ Cats
☐ Dog
☐ Bird
☐ Other furry

Figure 6.2 *Example of paediatric asthma admission pro-forma. Developed by the Brighton Paediatric Asthma Research Team, Royal Alexandra Hospital for Sick Children, Brighton. (Reproduced with permission.)*

(Back)

Current medication:

Date Started	Drug	Dose mcg/mg	Device/route	Frequency

Treatment of this attack at home

Drug	Dose mcg/mg	Route	Date/Time given

Examination details

Temp:.......... Pulse:......... Resps:......... PEF: Pre Bronchodilator.......... Post Bronchodilator:...............

Weight:........ Height:........ Oxygen sat: Pre Bronchodilator.......... Post Bronchodilator...............

Chest deformity:
- ☐ Yes
- ☐ No

Hyperinflated:
- ☐ Yes
- ☐ No

Accessory muscle use:
- ☐ Yes
- ☐ No

Cyanosis:
- ☐ Yes
- ☐ No

O2 Given?
- ☐ Yes
- ☐ No

Wheeze:
- ☐ Absent
- ☐ Audible normal breathing
- ☐ Audible deep breathing
- ☐ Audible without a stethoscope

Crackles:
- ☐ Left
- ☐ Right
- ☐ None

Recession:
- ☐ No
- ☐ Mild
- ☐ Moderate
- ☐ Severe

Air entry:
- ☐ Normal
- ☐ Left reduced
- ☐ Right reduced
- ☐ General reduction

Tracheal displacement:
- ☐ None
- ☐ Left
- ☐ Right

Apex beat displacement:
- ☐ None
- ☐ Left
- ☐ Right

Pulsus paradoxus:
- ☐ Present
- ☐ Absent

Nebuliser response:
- ☐ None
- ☐ Moderate
- ☐ Minimal
- ☐ Excellent

Other Examination:

Plan:
☐ Admit ☐ Home

Ward:
☐ Taaffe ☐ Cawthorne ☐ Nicholson ☐ Lydia

Impression/Management:

Figure 6.2 *(Continued).*

145

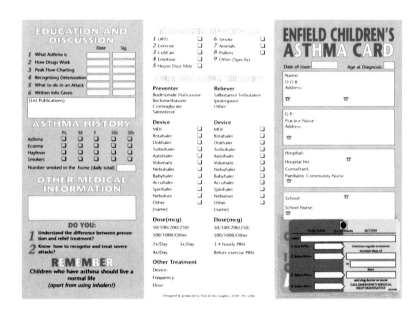

Figure 6.3 *Patient-held record card for asthma in childhood designed by the Enfield Children's Asthma Coordinating Committee. (Reproduced with permission from Dr Ian Pollock, Consultant Paediatrician, Chase Farm Hospital, EN2 8JL.)*

0910

CORNWALL & ISLES OF SCILLY
DISTRICT & FAMILY HEALTH SERVICE
AUTHORITIES

Asthma Referral Slip

From GP/ PN/ ALN/ SN/ DN/ HV/ CH/ AH/ PH.
To GP/ PN/ ALN/ SN/ DN/ HV/ CH/ PH
PLEASE CIRCLE

Acute Hospital ....
Community Hospital ....

GP General Practitioner PN Practice Nurse HV Health Visitor
SN School Nurse DN District Nurse PH Pharmacy
CH Community Hospital AH Acute Hospital
ALN Asthma Liason Nurse

I am referring Mr/Mrs/Ms .... Age ....
Address ....
for the following reason(s):

- Hospital Admission ☐ Attendance ☐
- Increase in use of bronchodilator ☐
- Evidence of increasing wheeze/cough ☐
- Prophylactic inhaler Rx not dispensed ☐
- Nocturnal/early morning symptoms ☐
- Poor compliance with prophylactic therapy ☐
- Poor inhaler technique ☐
- Side effects of medication ☐
- Requesting inappropriate OTC medication ☐
- Other comments ☐

Signature ....Date ....

Follow up in ......Days........Weeks.......Months

Other ....

CORNWALL & ISLES OF SCILLY
DISTRICT & FAMILY HEALTH SERVICE
AUTHORITIES

To be completed by GP/Nurse

Date of Consultation ....

Outcome

1. Counselling/education given on:
   - a) Compliance ☐
   - b) Inhaler Technique ☐
   - c) Self Management ☐
   - d) Avoidance of trigger factors ☐
2. Change of treatment
   From ....
   To ....
   Other details ....
   ....
3. Change of device
   From ....
   To ....
   Other details ....
   ....
4. Nebulised
5. Oral Steroids
6. Other advice/action taken ....
   ....

To be retained by P/N for audit purposes.

Figure 6.4 *Example of an acute asthma book. (Reproduced with kind permission from Mary White, Asthma Facilitator in Cornwall & Isles of Scilly Health Authorities.)*

Poor attendance at out-patients' departments for follow-up after acute attacks, coupled with high reattendance rates for uncontrolled asthma, justifies a new approach for caring for these patients. Attendance at casualty provides a unique opportunity for discussion and providing advice for those patients not deemed severe enough for admission. A trained nurse could provide this service and act as a link for communicating the details of the attendance to the primary care team[36].

Improving follow-up of patients recently admitted

After an acute asthma attack, many patients do not attend follow-up attendance at hospital. Why this happens, is unknown; however, it is worth speculating on some possibilities.

Shared care for asthma

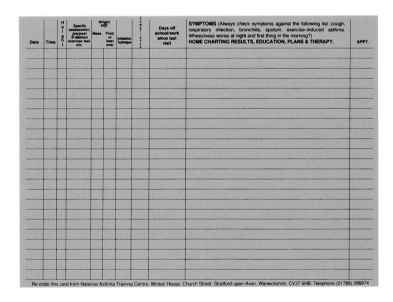

Figure 6.5 *National Asthma and Respiratory Training Centre card, available for sale from the NARTC, Warwick. (Reproduced with permission).*

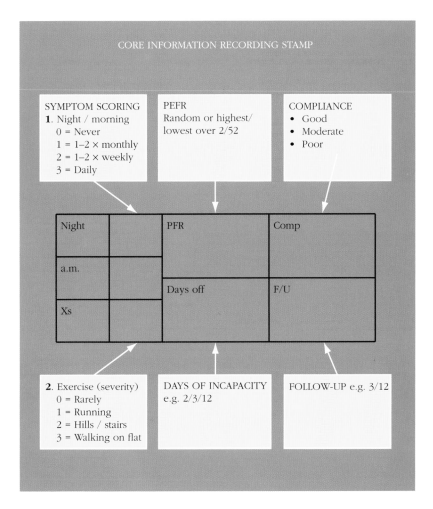

Figure 6.6 *Core information recording stamp (Dundee stamp). (Source: Tayside Asthma Group. Reproduced with permission).*

■ Having recovered from an acute attack, patients may feel well, possibly even a bit elated after a short course of oral prednisolone. This sense of well-being may engender a false sense of security explaining the patient's failure to return for follow-up.

149

- The follow-up appointment may have been arranged after an unacceptably long interval (for the patient) after the admission, by which time the patient may feel well or has forgotten the trauma of the attack.

Provision of follow-up care may be improved in a number of ways. GPs and trained asthma nurses should follow up most of these patients. Good, rapid communication from the hospital detailing the events leading up to and the treatment in hospital would facilitate this process. Appropriate follow-up arrangements after an acute attack should be included in any protocol for managing these attacks[18]. Those brittle or severe patients deemed to require hospital follow-up should be seen soon and preferably by an experienced doctor or nurse trained in asthma care.

Use of a specialist asthma nurse reduced reattendance for severe acute asthma as well as readmissions during 13 months following admission to a children's ward in Glasgow[25]. This was a randomized controlled study in which the intervention patients (children over 2 years old) were provided with an education booklet, a self-management plan, a course of oral steroids, a review discussion on the ward and a follow-up appointment in the nurses-run clinic two weeks later. This system of nurse-led discharge planning confirmed the benefit for the patients in terms of morbidity as well as reduced subsequent demand on hospital resources following acute asthma attacks in children.

Another study (Figure 6.7) recruited 211 adult patients attending A&E for asthma in a randomized controlled fashion[36]. Trained asthma nurses saw 80% of the intervention group at least once within six weeks of attending hospital. Less than 50% of this group attended the three appointments offered. The intervention in this study included a structured consultation by a nurse, involving an assessment of the severity of the patients' asthma, their medication and inhaler technique. All patients were provided with a written, personalized self management plan (see Figure 5.12) and taught how to recognize and manage attacks appropriately. After entry to the study, 35(33%) of active vs 45(42%) control patients had severe attacks (61 and 70, respectively, NS) during the six months. The intervention group reported (telephone interview) that they increased their use of inhaled topical steroids and rescue medication significantly more frequently in severe attacks than in the case of the controls. Six months after entry the intervention group had significantly higher and less variable peak flow and significantly lower and less variable symptom scores than the controls on their one week diary charts[36].

Educating patients

Most people who die from asthma have recently suffered a severe attack[47,48]. Therefore, patients need to understand why their asthma went out of control and how this could have been prevented. Then they may be in a position to prevent a future attack. Patients, like the rest of us, learn by example; therefore, our management of the acute attack serves as a role model for future episodes. If doctors do not use peak flow measurements or systemic steroids during the attack[1,27,42,48], how can patients be expected to do so in the future? (For more details on patient education and self-management plans, see Chapter 5.)

Those patients who make repeated use of A&E departments for their asthma management may be targeted for different, perhaps more intensive, follow-up. GPs may not be aware of these patients' repeated use of A&E departments. This is particularly a problem in large group practices where patients may not see the same doctor each time they attend. Therefore, the doctor reading the daily post, may not be aware that A&E reports therein relate to repeated attendances. It is important to try and identify and follow up these patients. In A&E departments this may be facilitated in the UK by the use of the unique NHS numbers. With computer systems, these repeat attendees may be identified and appropriate follow-up plans may then be made. GPs could incorporate similar systems in their practices, perhaps by drawing each emergency asthma attendance/discharge notification from hospital, to the attention of the practice nurse. The nurse could then carefully examine the records looking for previous hospital notifications and recall the patient for appropriate follow-up.

ASTHMA SELF-MANAGEMENT STUDY

Funded by the

Department of Medicine (Respiratory Unit),
Wellhouse NHS Trust, Wellhouse Lane,
Barnet EN5 3DJ. Telephone: 081 440 5111

Investigator   : Dr Mark Levy
Consultant Physicians   : Dr RJD Winter and Dr JC Bradley
Research Assistant   : Mrs Monica Robb
Asthma Research Nurses : Jo Allen and Carmel Doherty

NATIONAL **ASTHMA** CAMPAIGN
getting your breath back

ASTHMA CONSULTATION ON ___/___/___ : COPY FOR GENERAL PRACTITIONER & ASTHMA NURSE

Doctor_____   Research Number_____

_____   Re:

_____

As you know your patient has agreed to help in our study (approved by the District Ethics Committee) investigating the role of specialist asthma nurses in advising patients with a self management plan. This was the _____ of three visits and the consultation is summarised below. We have / previously enclosed a copy of the self management plan agreed with your patient. The nurses are working according to the recent Guidelines for adults circulated to all GP's in the UK. (Thorax supplement March 1993).

Date of recent A & E attendance___/___/____   Time attended: ____ : ___ hrs

Asthma Treatment   before attending A & E :   (Step **0 1 2 3 4 5**)

_____;____bd /tds/qds/prn	_____	Device
_____;____bd /tds/qds/prn	_____	Device
_____;____bd /tds/qds/prn	_____	Device
_____;____bd /tds/qds/prn	_____	Device
_____;____bd /tds/qds/prn	_____	Device

Patient contacted or saw GP before attending: Yes / No

   If yes:- did GP refer patient to hospital?   Yes / No

   If no :- did patient try to contact GP?   Yes / No

Time delay before attending A & E (since onset of symptoms)   __.__ Days (hours/24)

Was patient previously given a written self management plan?   Yes / No

Did patient try self management plan (SMP) before attending A&E?   Yes / No

IF YES:	Increased bronchodilator	Increased Inhaled steroid	Added Oral Steroid	Measured peak flow rate

Reason for attending A & E?   acute asthma / ran out of medication / other:...................

Outcome of A&E attendance? Sent Home / Admitted (Date discharged: ___/ ___/ ___)

After leaving hospital - Did patient attend the surgery?   Yes / No

   If Yes: saw GP / Nurse / Reception :   If Yes:- Was this for a prescription   Yes / No
       How many days after leaving hospital did patient attend?   __.__ Days (hours/24)

Figure 6.7(a,b)   A form used by respiratory nurses consulted by adult patients after attending the A&E department for an acute asthma episode. This form is used both as a means of communication (copies for hospital and general practice records) and in order to collect data for audit and research[36].

Assessment of asthma control since attending hospital:

Current treatment: (Step 0 1 2 3 4 5) ***

_____ ; ____	bd /tds/qds/prn _____	Device
_____ ; ____	bd /tds/qds/prn _____	Device
_____ ; ____	bd /tds/qds/prn _____	Device
_____ ; ____	bd /tds/qds/prn _____	Device
_____ ; ____	bd /tds/qds/prn _____	Device

Troublesome symptoms during the last week:

Cough : daytime : night : exertional   **Wheeze** : daytime ; night : exertional

Chest tightness : daytime ; night : exertional   **Chest pain** : daytime ; night : exertional

Other _____ : daytime ; night : exertional   dull : stabbing : constant : pressure

Need for relief medication }
since attending A & E: }   Daily : 2-3 times weekly : weekly : < weekly

Peak flow: Keeping a diary card?   **Yes / No**
                        If yes: Regularly / intermittently / never
                        If no : no meter / not been advised to / been advised to

   Usual best or predicted reading: _____ l/min

   Reading today: _____ l/min before bronchodilator   **% Predicted = __ %**

                   _____ l/min after bronchodilator   **Variability = __ %**

   Variability from peak flow diary: ___ % (during last week)

Inhaler type: Autohaler / Diskhaler / MDI / Rotahaler / Spinhaler / Turbohaler / Spacer / Nebuliser / Haleraid

Inhaler technique: Preparation ---> 	adequate /inadequate

                Expiration ---> 	adequate /inadequate = ___ **out of 4**

                Inspiration ---> 	adequate /inadequate

                Holds breath --> 	adequate /inadequate

Management plan: (Step 0 1 2 3 4 5)

1) Continue on current treatment as above *** using a _____ new device / as before.

2) Medication step change: We have replaced the _____ with _____ puffs

___ times daily, using a _____ device.

3) Self management action levels _____ (80%) _____ (60%) ____ (40%) **(see enclosed plan)**

4) **We advised the patient to consult you or your nurse for** _____.

Appointment given for ___/___/__ ; no more appointments given.

Seen by Sister Carmel Doherty / Sister Jo Allen: signed _____.

   (952 2381 bleep 621)   (440 5111 bleep 299)   therepdr.vr2

Figure 6.7 (Continued).

There are some brittle asthmatics well known to the hospital service who tend to go out of control quickly and where urgent admission to a respiratory or intensive care unit may be life-saving. Agreement should be made between the hospital service and the patient's GP regarding the course of action to be taken in each of these cases. The patient requires appropriate drug treatment and clear written self-management plans for emergencies and must know how to summon urgent help. In addition the ambulance service, A&E departments and respiratory wards need to have details of these patients and guidelines indicating how to handle them in an emergency. Ideally, the patient should have a shared-care card with details of their current and previous treatment.

Direct-access admission for adult asthma sufferers was pioneered by the respiratory service based at the Northern General Hospital in Edinburgh[1]. Crucial to the success of that service was the attachment of ventilatory facilities to the unit, staffed jointly between the anaesthetists and the respiratory physicians. The unit provided a pure respiratory service with no general medical commitment. It was well staffed with doctors and nurses trained in the assessment and management of acute severe asthma and able to perform endotracheal intubation and initiate ventilation. There is no doubt that it was successful in meeting the needs of the brittle asthmatics in its catchment area. However, such facilities are not available in most district general hospitals, where the approach often has to be more pragmatic. Rationalization of acute medical services within many NHS Hospital Trusts has meant many specialist respiratory facilities have been merged into General Medicine. As a consequence a number of respiratory physicians have now modified their admission policy for hot-line cases and have made arrangements for them to be seen initially in A&E departments where they may be assessed and stabilized before admission to the appropriate area. Fortunately, with improvements in general asthma care, the number of patients requiring these facilities is becoming less.

The need to ventilate a child with asthma is uncommon and the risk of a child dying from asthma is extremely low. Therefore it would be more appropriate to arrange direct access specifically for those children who are prone to very severe attacks of asthma. Children with acute asthma are more likely to present to the A&E department where detailed protocols for management should be available.

Ongoing audit and feedback

Many valuable opportunities for communication amongst colleagues are lost when information about patients is not shared. High quality feedback, from hospital to the GP and vice versa, about a patient's recent attendance, may be helpful. Hospital specialists may incorporate, in their discharge letters, information regarding appropriateness of the recent referral. GPs, on the other hand, could inform consultants when they feel that patients have been discharged too soon, as evidenced by persisting symptoms or even requests to revisit the patient out of hours soon after being discharged. Indeed these details could usefully be incorporated in pro-forma discharge letters, perhaps with a tear-off strip at the bottom for the GP to provide feedback to the hospital. In this way audit could become part

---

BTS audit criteria for patients treated for acute asthma in hospital[18]

- Admission PEF?
- Arterial blood gases if SaO_2 <92%?
- Systemic steroids administered? If so, how soon after arriving in hospital?
- PEF variability?
- Discharge prescription (inhaled and oral steroids)?
- Follow-up arrangements?
- Provision of self-management plan?

of the routine process of communication and form a focus for discussion at joint postgraduate education meetings.

The new British Guidelines on asthma care provide examples of audit criteria that could be incorporated into local audit systems[18].

Improving communications

With the establishment of NHS Trusts and Boards, pressures have been applied to increase the through-put of patients and to discharge them earlier. The BTS Guidelines suggest that patients should not be discharged unless the peak flow is >75% of predicted or best known, with a diurnal variation of <25% and no nocturnal symptoms[15,16,18]. However, due to pressure on acute services, this may be neither practical nor desirable in every instance. The BTS Audit showed that patients discharged with a diurnal PEF variation >25% were at increased risk of readmission to hospital[15]. Depending on the level of understanding of the patient and availability of asthma management within the patient's general practice, many may be discharged earlier, provided appropriate follow-up has been arranged with the primary care team. There is a need for discussions between hospital and primary care services to agree local policies. There may need to be different arrangements with different practices depending on their expertise in the management of asthma. If the practice has an established asthma clinic then a telephone call or fax notifying them of the early discharge followed by a letter with details of the hospital treatment and advice given should be made. Written instructions instructing patients how to manage their asthma and when to return to the ward should there be any problems would also be helpful.

Efficient communication from the hospital to the GP is extremely important. Any hospital doctor who doubts this fact should examine the criteria that purchasers require from provider units. Letters or discharge summaries should be sent promptly to the GP and be legible (preferably typewritten).

Many hospital doctors do not appreciate that a patient seen in the out-patient clinic, A&E department, or the person whom they have admitted under their care, may contact the GP within a few days of the visit to the hospital. The GP requires basic information about the hospital visit: this can either be handed to the patient, posted or, increasingly in the age of information technology, sent by fax or modem.

The information in the letter from the hospital should be clear, succinct and relevant to the GP or asthma nurse. Semi-structured letters, using clearly headed brief paragraphs and short phrases are better than long essays, however polished the prose. The information to be included within a discharge letter is detailed below and information to be provided by the GP to the hospital when asking for a patient to be admitted are listed on the following page. Examples of letters are given in Chapter 7.

Consider what information the GP will want? Sections giving details of the diagnosis, precisely what treatment has been prescribed or recommended, and follow-up arrangements are vital. If the GP's treatment has been altered, the reason for this should be explained. A brief description of the symptoms, signs on examination and, if appropriate, investigations should also be included. If there are concerns about the patient's or parents' understanding or compliance with treatment, these should be included. Details of any patient education, such as checking inhaler technique or giving a written self-management plan, should also be described.

Hospital discharge information urgently required by the general practitioner for further management

- Is this patient on oral steroids? If so, what dose, and when and how to stop.
- Has prophylactic medication been started or increased?
- Have there been any other changes from pre-attack medication?
- What was the result of the inhaler assessment? Best PEF?
- Details of the education provided, e.g. written self management plans.
- An indicator of trigger factor leading to admission, if known.
- What follow-up arrangements have been made?

Important information to be provided by the general practitioner when admitting a patient to hospital with an acute severe asthma attack

Clinical state at the time of initial assessment
- ability to speak or feed
- pulse rate
- respiratory rate
- peak expiratory flow + best achievable if known
- conscious level (in adults)

Measures taken to treat the patient
- corticosteroids given — dose and how administered
- beta agonists given — dose and how administered (nebulizer, inhaler plus spacer or by injection).
- ipratropium bromide or aminophylline given
- concentration of oxygen prescribed in ambulance

Regular drug therapy (including dose) before acute attack, and whether the patient adhered to this regime

Trigger factor if known or suspected

Social background, and relevant home environmental factors

Past medical history, particularly depression or psychosis.

Long-term maintenance and follow-up
The current situation

Long-term maintenance and follow-up care varies considerably across primary and secondary care sectors. Although many general practices provide organized asthma care (either in the form of set clinic times, or intermingled with the general medical and nursing service) about 20% of the nurses providing the care are inadequately trained[26]. Hospital care of asthmatics may not always be provided by those with experience in this field.

Most childhood asthma is managed in primary care. However, asthma is the commonest chronic childhood condition treated in hospital and it could be argued that all paediatricians should be trained to manage these children. This argument is strengthened by the fact that there are extremely few specialist respiratory paediatricians to whom GPs and general paediatricians can refer their children who suffer from complicated forms of asthma.

Adult asthma clinics are uncommon in hospital units other than tertiary units. The standard of provision of chronic follow-up for adult asthmatic patients varies considerably. In some units a specialist with an interest in respiratory disease may see all asthmatics while in others this work may be delegated to junior doctors without much experience.

Improving monitoring and follow-up

Setting up an asthma clinic in primary care: A number of personnel are employed within the practice setting and asthma management is but one part in their complex interreaction.

The development of a practice protocol for asthma management may enhance teamwork and ensure that consistent advice is given to patients. Aide memoirs, perhaps modified from the practice protocol or national guidelines[18], in each consulting room covering the salient points of the assessment and management plans may be helpful. While a practice may have a doctor and/or practice nurse particularly interested in, and charged with, the management of the asthma service, it is essential that all staff have relevant understanding and education so that appropriate action can be taken, irrespective of who is 'on call' if an emergency arises (Figure 6.8) (see also Chapter 7).

The logistics involved in setting up[3,20–22,50–54] and evaluating[21,22,52,55] nurse-run asthma clinics have been well described elsewhere and this aspect is dealt with only in outline in this book.

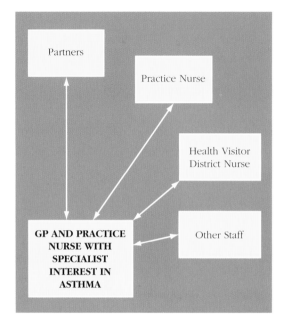

Figure 6.8
Interrelationships in the primary care team.

Having decided to set up a nurse-run asthma clinic, the first priority is to ensure appropriate training for the personnel involved. Attendance by nurses and doctors on one of the comprehensive asthma training courses, in combination with in-house training, is probably the best place to start. The facilities required include:

- consulting rooms
- protected time with provision for the nurse to communicate effectively with the doctor
- record-keeping facilities and the maintenance of an asthma register
- peak flow meters and spirometry equipment, placebo inhaler devices and teaching aids for demonstration
- diary cards for patients
- arrangements for organizing follow-up (including identification of non-attendees) and communication between other health professionals (community and hospital) involved in the care of these patients.

Levels of practice nurse involvement in asthma clinics

Minimum role — patient always sees GP
Clinic tasks
1. Compiling asthma register
2. Taking a structured formal history
3. Taking peak flows in surgery
4. Teaching how to use peak flow meter at home, and how to chart a diary card
5. Demonstrating, instructing, checking inhaler technique

Medium role — potential for a GP/Nurse clinic
Clinic tasks (1–5) plus
6. Carrying out further tests, e.g. reversibility, exercise
7. Improving asthma education
8. Providing explanatory literature
9. Spotting poor control, with referral back to GP
10. Establishing regular follow-up procedure

Maximum role/autonomy — nurse-run clinic with GP availability
Clinic tasks (1–10) plus
11. Carrying out full assessments and regular follow-up
12. Formulating structured treatment plan in conjunction with GP + patient
13. Preparing prescriptions for approval by GP
14. Giving telephone advice where appropriate
15. Seeing patients first in an 'emergency', i.e. a presentation with increased or renewed symptoms.

(Reproduced with permission from the National Asthma and Respiratory Training Centre (NARTC), Warwick.)

Clear boundaries have to be set in defining the nurse's role, which should depend on their training and experience. In many areas there are asthma nurses who are qualified trainers and advisers. They could give appropriate support and guidance to less qualified colleagues through the setting up of nurse groups that meet and support each other regularly. It is essential that the nurse involved in the asthma service is supported and this includes having doctors available to help deal with difficult problems[24].

Patient education and treatment modification: Patient education will help to improve compliance and can involve asthma resource centres, respiratory liaison nurses and schools.

Patient education is not simply a one-way transfer of information from clinician to patient. Evans[35] suggests that while this aspect of education is important, patients need to overcome three broad obstacles before they can manage to control their asthma adequately. The following paragraphs are based strongly on Evans' article in *Thorax*[35] (with permission).

■ Patients need to understand what asthma means on a personal level.

Personal feelings, such as anger, self-blame, fear, lessened self-esteem, and beliefs about asthma (e.g. that it increases vulnerability, that it is an acute rather than a chronic disease, or that it is a psychological illness) may influence a newly diagnosed asthmatic patients' adherence to medical advice. Evans suggests that clinicians are often unaware of these beliefs. One of the aims of the consultation should be to 'to discover what the patient's knowledge, beliefs and feelings about asthma are, to reinforce those that are appropriate and accurate, and to begin the process of persuading the patient to change those that are not'.

■ Patients need to acquire information and skills needed to prevent and control asthma.

This task includes recognizing and responding to symptoms of asthma, understanding the purposes of different types of medicines, learning to use them correctly, and making appropriate decisions about when to seek emergency care. The correct use of an inhaler is complex and those caring for asthmatic patients need to familiarize themselves thoroughly with their use, before teaching patients.

■ Patients must learn to manage key relationships so that they and their family can live normal, active lives.

For parents of children with asthma, this means learning to talk with schoolteachers to get support for carrying out the child's treatment plan at school, or managing family relationships to minimize disruption of activities or relationships with siblings. For children, it means learning to explain asthma to peers and to overcome teasing or exclusion from games. For adults with asthma it may involve talking with employers about controlling environmental irritants and using asthma medicines in the workplace. These issues are often critical to the success of a preventive treatment strategy.

Much has been written on the failure of patients to adhere to medical advice and to attend for follow-up appointments. Human nature dictates that people will seek medical assistance when they are unwell. Therefore, perhaps health professionals need to focus their attention on patients when they attend with uncontrolled asthma **and** other medical or even administrative problems, such as for medical certificates, reports and disabled car badges.

Patient education doesn't simply involve demonstration of inhaler technique[35]. When patients or parents are told the diagnosis of asthma, this has different implications for each person. If they are immediately bombarded with asthma education and self-management plans, it is unlikely that they will be compliant, because they have not yet come to terms with the diagnosis. Perhaps we can draw some parallels from the literature on bereavement[57]. At the moment of hearing the diagnosis of asthma, the person's life changes. This is likely to be met with strong feelings of denial and an emotional numbness: one can almost hear the patient saying 'this can't be happening to me'. The doctor may think the patient is very calm and rational, but the patient may feel 'mummified'. Later, other feelings follow: grief, anger, depression, guilt. This might not happen in the doctor's surgery, but at home. Finally, the person or the family begin to accept what they have been told and to make the necessary practical adjustments to their lives. There is no way of predicting how long this process will take, but education and self-management may have to be delayed until the person has accepted the diagnosis. Therefore a *whole person approach* is required in order to deal with patient expectations and anxieties, and provide adequate information related to asthma, its management and early recognition of impending attacks.

An innovative approach has been developed in one area. Dr Mike Ward (personal communication) and his team in Sutton-in-Ashfield, UK, provide ongoing care and education in their asthma resource centre. This centre is housed in an accessible, separate building from the main hospital, staffed by specially trained nurses, and patients may attend when they wish, either with or without an appointment.

In areas where general practitioner asthma clinics are well developed, a centre for asthma may be underused. However, in other areas where the standard of asthma management may be lower or for specific problem groups, such as teenagers, open-access clinics would be worth exploring.

Hospital specialist respiratory nurses: An important development in recent years has been the appointment of an increasing number of hospital-based, respiratory specialist nurses. These nurses should have more time and if properly trained, may be able to communicate appropriate information to patients. Good communication between the hospital and practice nurses could improve the management of patients requiring shared care, particularly following admission for an attack. A dialogue between the hospital and primary care may facilitate development of joint protocols and enable appropriate training of respiratory liaison nurses similar to that for practice nurses.

Childhood asthma and schools: There are a number of important issues related to childhood asthma and schools (Figure 6.9):

- In a class of 30 there may be up to six children suffering from asthma
- Many teachers have a limited understanding of asthma and are often frightened of it
- There is reluctance in some schools for teachers to be involved in the management of the asthmatic child, i.e. administration of medication
- Many children are not allowed by the school to carry and administer their own medication according to their self-management plans. We believe this is wrong and suggest that children who are able should be able to carry out their own medication
- Owing to the widespread availability of the National Asthma Campaign's Schools Pack, many schools have raised their staff awareness of asthma. However, very few schools have emergency medication (reliever inhalers) available for use if a child has an attack. The authors believe this situation should change.

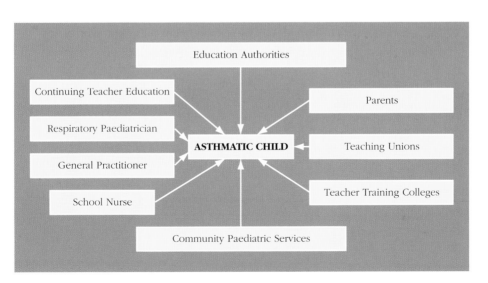

Figure 6.9 *People influencing management of the child at school.*

Education authorities should be encouraged to adapt an agreed policy for the management of the asthmatic children in their care and to ensure that childhood asthma has a prominent place in the Teacher Training College and continuing teacher education curriculum. Discussions need to take place with teachers' unions to allay fears of their members and encourage the teachers' involvement in the management of the child while at school. Paediatricians, including the Community Paediatric Services, School Nurses and GPs need to be actively involved in this process at a local level. In Scotland all the education authorities have been approached by, and have asked for, the SIGN schools asthma initiative, made up of representatives of the above professional groups, to work with them to draw up such protocols.

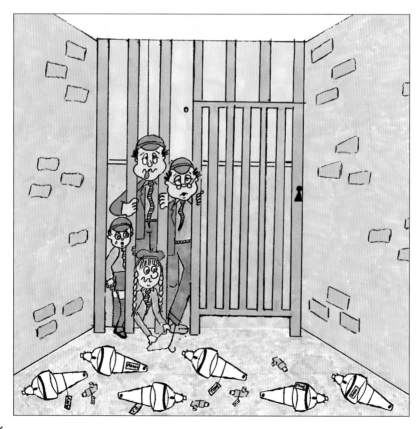

Recently the Community Paediatric Service has been undergoing a major reorganization. As part of this process the training programme has been re-examined to make it more appropriate to the needs of the service. This is being done at a local level and it is important that paediatricians and GPs with an interest in childhood asthma should have an input, to ensure that the teaching of asthma management appears in the new curriculum, particularly as this service is ideally placed to monitor the management of asthma in schools and provide appropriate advice and education to the School Health Service.

In difficult cases, dialogue between the GP and the child's school should be encouraged to facilitate appropriate management. In an emergency, schools should be encouraged to seek medical advice from the primary care team or hospital services without waiting for parental consent.

Non-attenders in primary care: In primary care, nurse-run asthma clinics are clearly beneficial for those patients who attend (otherwise they wouldn't!) and are providing a perceived need. However, a different approach is needed for those patients who fail to respond to

---

Resources for asthma care and education in schools

■ The National Asthma Campaign has produced School Packs for staff with relevant information on the disease, management and recognition of acute attacks.

■ The National Asthma and Respiratory Training Centre has produced excellent teaching materials to answer teachers' questions and address their anxieties about asthma.

■ The School Asthma Card is useful for summarizing treatment information and contact phone numbers in the case of emergencies (Figure 6.10).

■ Control Your Asthma — a card produced jointly by the NAC and the Department of Health.

Card checked

Date	Initials

NATIONAL **ASTHMA** CAMPAIGN
getting your breath back

School asthma card

Name

Address

Telephone	Home
	Parent's work

| General | Name |
| Practitioner | Telephone |

Consultant

Hospital	Name
	Reference number
	Telephone

Providence House
Providence Place
London N1 0NT

Facsimile
071 704 0740

If you would like
a copy of the pamphlet
Asthma at school please
write to the address above.

4

**This card is for your school.
Remember to update it if treatment
is changed.**

1

**Regular treatment to be
taken in school time**

Name and how taken	Dose and when taken

Before exercise

_____

_____

_____

2

**Relief treatment
when needed**

For sudden chest tightness,
wheeze, breathlessness or
cough, give or allow child
to take

Name and how taken	Dose and when taken

If no relief or symptoms reappear within three hours

- Repeat above
- Call parent

If child is fighting for breath, speechless or blue

- Repeat above
- Call parent
- Dial 999 for an ambulance
  or
- take to nearest hospital

3

Figure 6.10 *NAC school asthma card.*

invitations to attend. One of the ways of identifying non-attenders may be through the repeat prescribing system, where patients may request prescriptions without seeing the doctor. Most surgeries have these systems in place and all have different ways of identifying when patients need to attend for review. For example, if six prescriptions (i.e. 6-months' worth) have been issued, the patient will be asked to attend before any more are issued. By strictly adhering to a system like this, patients would have to attend at least every 6 months. An analogous situation is the provision of contraceptive prescriptions where patients have to attend for blood pressure estimation every 6 months before a new prescription is issued.

Telephone advice and monitoring has been fairly successful in some studies. In a randomized controlled study[36] of provision of asthma care for adults following attendance at an A&E department for an attack, patients' symptoms, peak flow measurements and adjustment of therapy were discussed on the telephone with those unwilling to attend in person. The nurses found that it was possible to conduct a useful telephone educational consultation with these patients.

Involvement of reception staff: Due to a lack of training, receptionists may be unaware of the dangers of uncontrolled asthma and the need for urgent intervention by the patient, the family and the health professionals. Provided sufficient information is given when the patient telephones or attends for an urgent consultation, most asthmatic exacerbations can be dealt with efficiently and quickly. This may be achieved by:

- improving understanding and knowledge of the receptionists;
- teaching patients what information to provide when seeking help (see box). (Perhaps this information could be incorporated into the patient's self management plan.)

> **What patients need to say to receptionists when requesting urgent consultations for asthma**
>
> ■ Say that you/your child have asthma and that it is out of control.
> ■ Explain that you/your child have been advised to consult the nurse or doctor when you/your child's asthma goes out of control.
> ■ Tell the receptionist if you/your child have needed to use extra relief medication.
> ■ Tell the receptionist if you/your child's asthma has been waking you/your child from sleep.

Referral to hospital and communication across the interface:
Who should be referred to hospital?

Whether a GP decides to refer a child for a specialist opinion depends not only on the child's symptoms and the parents' concerns and expectations, but also on the doctor's experience of childhood asthma and confidence in dealing with the illness. It is evident that many practices have a particular interest in asthma and provide a very high standard of care. Such practices often follow nationally or locally agreed guidelines for asthma management; they often have asthma clinics run by a trained practice nurse who reviews children's treatment regularly at planned intervals. Hospital referrals from such practices are infrequent and occur only if the child meets certain criteria for seeking a specialist opinion (see box).

At the other end of the spectrum, there are GPs who are not confident enough to make a firm diagnosis of asthma, to start appropriate treatment or to reassure the family. They may see children only during acute crises, when the asthma is unstable, and there are no planned regular reviews. Such practices have a low threshold for seeking a paediatric opinion, and refer a much higher proportion of their patients with asthma than other neighbouring

Hospital referral should be considered:[15]

Children
- If the diagnosis is in doubt
- If asthma is unstable
- If asthma is impairing normal activities
- For reassurance or support of parents or GP
- For those children needing > 400 µg/day inhaled steroids

Adults
- Occupational asthma, to establish the diagnosis
- If the diagnosis is in doubt
- For pregnant women with worsening asthma
- For patients with COPD and an asthmatic component who are not responding to treatment

practices. Many of the children they refer do not require hospital involvement.

The BTS guidelines[15] suggest that inadequate control of symptoms on >400 µg/day of an inhaled steroid is a reason for paediatric referral. Some GPs would question this criterion and it is doubtful whether the hospital sector could cope with the additional demand. A significant number of referrals are made because parents or the GPs themselves are seeking reassurance about either the diagnosis or the treatment that has been given. In particular, parents (and health professionals) are concerned about the safety of inhaled steroids.

In some children's departments, there are specialist respiratory paediatricians. They see children with complex chest disorders, including those with severe asthma, who are referred by general or community paediatricians and by GPs. Children who have had a single life-threatening episode of asthma, those who have severely restricted activities, such as prolonged periods off school because of their asthma, and those with brittle asthma, should be referred to such

171

Asthmatic patients who require follow-up by a respiratory specialist

Children

■ After a life-threatening episode
■ Children with very brittle asthma
■ Those whose activities are severely restricted
■ If special investigations are needed
■ Those children needing > 800 µg/day[15] inhaled steroids
■ Those requiring regular oral steroids
■ Those needing > four short courses of oral steroids a year

Adults

■ Patients with life-threatening asthma
■ Patients who require ventilation
■ Those who have developed complications or have recurrent severe attacks
■ Patients on long-term oral steroids
■ Those requiring regular nebulizer treatment
■ Those with significant social problems.

a specialist children's chest clinic. Children who require high doses of inhaled steroids, continuous oral steroids, or frequent short courses of oral steroids for acute exacerbations, may also benefit from being seen in a specialist clinic.

While most adult asthmatics should be managed in the community, it is sometimes necessary to seek specialist advice. We recommend referral of patients with suspected occupational asthma because this condition may be very difficult to diagnose, it attracts compensation and most importantly, this condition may resolve on reduced exposure to the offending allergen. Similarly referral is required if the diagnosis is in doubt.

Pregnant women with worsening asthma and patients with COPD and an asthmatic component who are not responding to treatment may benefit from specialist help.

Referral letter from GP to a hospital specialist

The information contained in the referral letter from the GP is usually the only information that the consultant has when the patient enters the clinic. A poor referral letter places both clinician and patient at an unnecessary disadvantage (see Chapter 7).

A brief history outlining the nature, frequency and severity of the symptoms, and the way in which they affect the patient and the family, is essential. The letter should contain brief details of previous illnesses, the need for short courses of oral steroids and hospital admissions. Precise details of current asthma therapy, what dose and which inhaler device is being used, are vital. 'Two puffs of Becotide bd' is unacceptably vague and guarantees confusion: does this mean $100\,\mu g$ bd, $400\,\mu g$ bd or $500\,\mu g$ bd?

The reason for the referral should be stated explicitly: is the GP seeking a one-off consultation to confirm that the management is appropriate, or to reassure anxious patients or parents who are demanding a second opinion, or does the GP want the specialist to take on the long-term care of the patient? What are the patient's, parents', child's and the doctor's anxieties and expectations? They may be quite different from each other. If the letter informs the specialist about family illnesses or stresses, this will influence the way the consultation is conducted: for example, knowing that a family member recently died of a respiratory disorder, or that a child is upset because the parents have recently separated, may be extremely important.

All these details can usually be covered on a single sheet of A4 paper or less (see Chapter 7).

Long-term follow-up of patients by the hospital service

Long-term follow-up needs to be discussed locally and will depend on the expertise and concerns of individual GPs and local respiratory physicians. It is often not feasible for the hospital to follow up all admissions within one month. It is better to be selective and involve cases that have given rise to concern where a respiratory consultant's input is helpful rather than to allow indiscriminate follow-up at SHO level. Hospital follow-up of adult patients should always be by a respiratory physician although it may not be feasible for a paediatrician with a respiratory interest to deal with all the problems in that area.

The Scottish Intercollegiate Guidelines Network (SIGN) subgroup has addressed issues involving working at the interface between hospital and general practice. They recommended that a patient's medication should be reviewed within two to four weeks after discharge following an acute attack. Following an asthma attack all patients need to be seen and kept under review until their asthma is under control and they have confidence in managing future attacks. Follow-up may occur at the hospital or in primary care, as long as it is provided by someone with an interest in, and knowledge of, asthma care[58]. While general practices with a well developed asthma care infrastructure may be happy to follow up most patients with acute severe asthma, there may be others who are less confident in asthma management and may well value input from the hospital service.

Standardizing prescribing policy: Medication for the management of asthma, particularly some of the newer drugs and devices can be expensive. The Health Boards in Scotland and Northern Ireland, the Health Authorities in England and Wales and the NHS Prescribing Unit try to influence general practice prescribing. This approach is largely aimed at reducing costs of prescribing and GPs often find themselves defending their overspends against criticism by medical advisers when they overspend. This aspect is discussed in Chapter 2[59].

In an effort to reduce costs, GPs are encouraged to use generic rather than brand name drugs; however, there are insufficient data to confirm that these products are equally effective[18]. Each practice needs to draw up its own formulary of approved drugs to be used in the management of asthma; this needs to be agreed and adhered to by all partners. Practical help in this respect may be available from Health Boards and Authorities who employ pharmaceutical advisers. Whilst the taking of inhaled steroids through a spacer device may be the first line of treatment, flexibility is important to allow the change to other medication or devices if initial treatment fails. It is important that the special needs of children are recognized when the practice formulary is devised.

Differences in prescribing patterns between hospitals and general practice may cause problems, particularly if the hospital doctors suggest expensive new medications as first-line treatment for a disease that is normally controllable by standard therapy. These drugs may be available to hospitals at discount prices. However, once they have been prescribed in the community, the GP has to bear the full cost of such medications. Until recently, hospital doctors have had considerably more leeway when prescribing expensive drugs, although they are now being held more accountable for their actions; in consequence they have become more aware of the problems faced by their GP colleagues. This is an area where discussions between all healthcare providers should be encouraged in order to develop joint protocols and formularies.

Establishing outreach clinics: The development of fund-holding practices has stimulated the question of outreach clinics. In some rural areas, such as the Highland Region, consultants have run clinics in remote areas for many years. This has resulted in improved communication, mutual education of health professionals as well as benefiting the outlying communities.

The idea that a fund-holding practice within an urban area may 'buy in' the services of a local physician, to see their general medical cases, including those with asthma, within the practice setting, is a relatively new concept and there is little information on the practicability and cost-effectiveness of this approach. The primary care team and the consultant need to develop a protocol for referral and management of patients. It is important that the total service provided at least matches that provided in the hospital setting. Outreach clinics may stimulate audit with subsequent improvement in the service across the interface of care. At present there are not enough physicians to provide all practices with these services and therefore in most cases the specialist consultation and assessment takes place within the hospital setting. With more asthma patients being treated in the community, outreach clinics may provide new opportunities for training health professionals as well as for implementing research.

Audit of ongoing care of asthma: Ongoing audit of care in the community and in hospital could provide a continuous method of providing feedback and training for health professionals. The latest version of the British Guidelines for asthma care provide some useful criteria for audit. Examples of these are shown in the boxes and figures in this chapter.

In summary, the message conveyed in this chapter is that clear communication is fundamental to the concept of effective integrated care. All those involved in asthma care need to listen carefully to their patients' concerns and expectations as well as to the opinions and feelings of all the health professionals involved. A consistent approach to management needs to be developed locally by health professionals.

References

1 British Thoracic Association. Death from asthma in two regions. *BMJ* 1982; **285**: 1251–5.

2 Modell M, Harding J, Horder E *et al.* Improving the care of asthmatics in general practice. *BMJ* 1983; **286**: 2027–30.

3 Pearson R, Barnes G. Asthma clinics in general practice. In: Levy M, ed. *Asthma in practice.* Exeter: Royal College of GPs, 1987; pp. 15–20.

4 Barnes GR. Nurse-run hypertension clinics. *J Roy Coll Gen Pract* 1983; **33**: 820–1.

5 Speight AN, Lee DA, Hey EN. Underdiagnosis and undertreatment of asthma in childhood. *Br Med J* 1983; **286**: 1253–6.

6 Anderson HR, Bailey PA, Cooper JS, Palmer JC, West S. Influence of morbidity illness label and social, family and health service factors on drug treatment of childhood asthma. *Lancet* 1981; **2**: 1030–2.

7 Heeijne Den Bak J. Prevalence and management of asthma in children under 16 in one practice. *BMJ* 1986; **292**: 175–6.

8 Toop LJ, Howie JGR, Paxton FM. Night cough and general practice research. *J Roy Coll Gen Pract* 1986; **290**: 76-7.

9 Tudor-Hart J. Wheezing in young children: problems of measurement and management. *J Roy Coll Gen Pract* 1986; **36**: 78–81.

10 Levy M, Parmar M, Coetzee D *et al*. Respiratory consultations in asthmatic compared with non-asthmatic children in general practice. *BMJ* 1985; **291**: 29–30.

11 Toop LJ. Active approach to recognising asthma in general practice. *BMJ* 1985; **290**: 1629–31.

12 Levy M, Bell L. General practice audit of asthma in childhood. *BMJ* 1984; **289**: 1115–16.

13 Levy M. The GPs in Asthma Group. *Prim Health Care Man* 1993; **3**: 10.

14 Anon. *Asthma*. Exeter, Devon: RCGP, 1987.

15 Anon. Guidelines on the management of asthma. Statement by the British Thoracic Society, the British Paediatric Association, the Research Unit of the Royal College of Physicians of London, the King's Fund Centre, the National Asthma Campaign, the Royal College of General Practitioners, the GPs in Asthma Group, the British Association of A&E Medicine and the British Paediatric Respiratory Group. *Thorax* 1993; **48**: S1–24. [Published errata appear in *Thorax* 1994; **49**: 96 and 1994; **49**: 386.]

16 British Thoracic Society *et al*. Guidelines for the management of asthma: a summary. *BMJ* 1993; **306**: 776–82.

17 British Thoracic Society. Guidelines for management of asthma in adults: II. Acute severe asthma. *BMJ* 1990; **301**: 797–800.

18 The British Thoracic Society, The National Asthma Campaign, The Royal College of Physicians of London, The GPs in Asthma Group, The British Association of A&E Medicine, The British Paediatric Respiratory Society, The British Guidelines on Asthma Management: 1995 Review and Position Statement. *Thorax* 1997; **52**(Suppl.): S1–21.

19 Neville RG, Hoskins G, Smith B *et al*. Observations on the structure, process and clinical outcomes of asthma care in general practice. *Br J Gen Pract* 1996; **46**: 583–7.

20 Levy M, Hilton S. The role of the practice nurse. In: *Asthma in practice*. London: RCGP, 1993; pp. 75–9.

21 Charlton I, Charlton G, Broomfield J, Campbell M. An evaluation of a nurse-run asthma clinic in general practice using an attitudes and morbidity questionnaire. *Fam Prac* 1992; **9**: 154–60.

22 Charlton I. Asthma clinics: audit. *Practitioner* 1989; **233**: 1522–3.

23 Taggart VS, Zuckerman AE, Lucas S, Acty-Lindsey A, Bellanti JA. Adapting a self-management education program for asthma for use in an outpatient clinic. *Ann Allergy* 1987; **58**: 173–8.

24 Barnes G. Nurse run asthma clinics in general practice. *J Roy Coll Gen Pract* 1985; **34**: 447.

25 Madge P, McColl J, Paton J. Impact of a nurse-led home management training programme in children admitted to hospital with acute asthma: a randomized controlled study. *Thorax* 1997; **52**: 223–8.

26 Barnes G, Partridge MR. Community asthma clinics: 1993 survey of primary care by the National Asthma Task Force. *Qual Health Care* 1994; **3**: 133–6.

27 Wright SC, Evans AE, Sinnamon DG, MacMahon J. Asthma mortality and death certification in Northern Ireland. *Thorax* 1994; **49**: 141–3.

28 Neville RG, Clark RC, Hoskins G, Smith B. National asthma attack audit 1991–2. GPs in Asthma Group [see Comments]. *BMJ* 1993; **306**: 559–62.

29 Stableforth DE. Asthma deaths in the UK. *New England and Regional Allergy Proceedings* 1993; **7**: 435–8.

30 Wareham NJ, Harrison BD, Jenkins PF, Nicholls J, Stableforth DE. A district confidential enquiry into deaths due to asthma. *Thorax* 1993; **48**: 1117–20.

31 Bucknall CE, Robertson C, Moran F, Stevenson RD. Improving management of asthma: closing the loop or progressing along the audit spiral? *Qual Health Care* 1992; **1**: 15–20.

32 Fletcher HJ, Ibrahim SA, Speight N. Survey of asthma deaths in the Northern region, 1970-85 [see Comments]. *Arch Dis Child* 1990; **65**: 163–7.

33 Bucknall CE, Robertson C, Moran F, Stevenson RD. Management of asthma in hospital: a prospective audit. *BMJ* 1988; **296**: 1637–9.

34 Bucknall CE, Robertson C, Moran F, Stevenson RD. Differences in hospital asthma management. *Lancet* 1988; **1**: 748–50.

35 Evans D. To help patients control asthma the clinician must be a good listener and teacher. *Thorax* 1993; **48**: 685–7.

36 Levy ML, Robb M, Allen J, Doherty C, Bland M, Winter RJD. Guided self-management reduces morbidity, time off work and consultations for uncontrolled asthma in adults. *Eur Resp J* 1995; Suppl. **19**: 318s.

37 Fitzgerald JM. Psychological barriers to asthma education. *Chest* 1994; **106**: 2605–35.

38 Costa Pereira ANR. *Asthma-like symptoms in the community: a study of care.* 1993; PhD Thesis, Dundee University.

39 Partridge MR, Latouche D, Trako E, Thurston JB. A national census of those attending UK A&E departments with asthma. *Eur Resp J* 1995; Suppl. **19**: 164s.

40 Levy ML, Robb M, Bradley JL, Winter RJD. Presentation and self management in acute asthma: a prospective study in two districts. *Thorax* 1993; **48**: 460–1.

41 Hilton SR, GPs in Asthma Group. General practice survey of acceptability and impact of the 1990 guidelines for management of adult asthma. *Thorax* 1991; **46**: 741p.

42 Eason J, Markowe HJL. Controlled investigation of deaths from asthma in hospitals in the North-East Thames region. *BMJ* 1987; **294**: 1255–8.

43 Pearson MG, Ryland I, Harrison BD, on behalf of the British Thoracic Society's Standards of Care Committee. National audit of acute severe asthma in adults admitted to hospital. *Qual Health Care* 1995; **4**: 24–30.

44 Town I, Kwong T, Holst P, Beasley R. Use of a management plan for treating asthma in an emergency department. *Thorax* 1990; **45**: 702–6.

45 White M, Waldron M. A study to assess the need for a referral book for patients with asthma. *Thorax* 1996; **51**: A62.

46 Connett GJ, Warde C, Wooler E *et al.* Audit strategies to reduce hospital admissions for acute asthma. *Arch Dis Child* 1993; **69**: 202–5.

47 Asthma Mortality Task Force 1986. American Academy of Allergy and Immunology and the American Thoracic Society. *J Allergy Clin Immunol* 1987; **80**: 361–514.

48 Rea HH, Scragg R, Jackson R, Beaglehole R, Fenwick J, Sutherland DC. A case-control study of deaths from asthma. *Thorax* 1986; **41**: 833–9.

49 Crompton GK. Edinburgh emergency asthma admission service: Report on 10 years' experience. *BMJ* 1979; **2**: 1199–207.

50 Charlton I. Asthma clinics: setting up. *Practitioner* 1989; **233**: 1359–60.

51 Charlton I. Asthma clinics: how to run one. *Practitioner* 1989; **233**: 1440–2,1445.

52 Charlton I, Charlton G, Broomfield J, Mullee MA. Audit of the effect of a nurse run asthma clinic on workload and patient morbidity in a general practice. *Br J Gen Pract* 1991; **41**: 227–31.

53 Unit 5 Patients, doctors and the practice nurse. In: *The distance learning pack for the NATC Diploma*. Stratford-upon-Avon: National Asthma Training Centre, 1995.

54 Pietroni R, Levy M. An interdisciplinary course on asthma and diabetes in general practice. *Postgrad Educ Gen Pract* 1992; **3**: 41–6.

55 Charlton I, Antoniou AG, Atkinson J *et al*. Asthma at the interface: bridging the gap between general practice and a district general hospital. *Arch Dis Child* 1994; **70**: 313–18.

56 Asthma clinics. In: *The distance learning pack for the NATC Diploma*. Stratford-upon-Avon: National Asthma Training Centre, 1995.

57 Worden JW. Attachment, loss, and the tasks of mourning. In: *Grief counselling and grief therapy*. London, New York: Tavistock Publications, 1987; pp. 7–18.

58 Scottish Intercollegiate Guidelines Network. Hospital In-Patient Management of Acute Asthma Attacks. 1996; **6**: 1–29.

59 Price DB. Inhaled steroid prescribing over seven years in a general practice and its implications. *Eur Resp J* 1995; (Suppl. 19): 463s.

Chapter 7

Case studies and examples of referral letters

Case studies

Case 1: A child with pet allergy

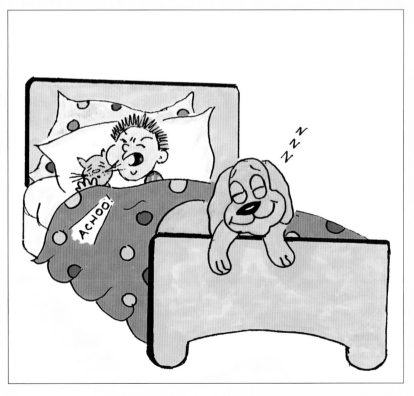

Danielle, a 12-year-old girl with chronic asthma, was referred to a children's chest clinic with persistent nocturnal cough, despite increasing doses of inhaled steroids and bronchodilators. On direct questioning, she said that the family's dog slept in her bedroom, despite the fact that when she played with the dog, she developed itchy eyes, sneezing, cough and wheeze. After the family were convinced that the hound should be banished from the bedroom, and the room was thoroughly cleaned, her symptoms reduced dramatically and it was possible to halve the dose of inhaled steroids.

Comment

A detailed history is the most important tool for diagnosing allergy. Increasing the preventative medication is not always the correct response to increasing symptoms. A home visit by the general practitioner, community or practice asthma nurse is sometimes helpful in establishing why a patient's asthma is difficult to control.

Case 2: Anxiety, overtreatment and the need for a multidisciplinary approach

David, a 13-year-old boy with severe asthma, was referred to a respiratory paediatrician by his general paediatrician. Despite prolonged treatment with increasing doses of inhaled steroids, salmeterol, theophylline and short-acting bronchodilators, he had missed a third of his schooling in the previous year. He felt unable to take part in the most minor of physical activities at school, home or socially. As a result of the continuous oral prednisolone he had received, he had become overtly cushingoid. At the time of referral, David was receiving 21 different medications for his asthma, eczema and allergic rhinitis. His mother presented the paediatrician with a computer print-out of his medications that she had produced.

On examination, he was cushingoid. His weight was on the 90th and his height below the 3rd centile for his age. There were no abnormalities in his chest. Spirometry was normal. Mother and child appeared to be very anxious about all the details of his asthma and its treatment.

Simplifying his complicated therapy produced no improvement over the next month. It seemed that further manipulation of his treatment was unlikely to be successful and that there were major psychological issues that needed to be dealt with. Telephone discussions with the GP, practice nurse and local paediatrician supported the view that both mother and child had become extremely nervous about any attempts to either decrease David's medication or to increase his level of activity. It was suggested to David and his mother that a period of in-patient care and observation might be helpful: rather surprisingly, this was enthusiastically agreed to by both of them.

On admission to the children's ward, David was withdrawn and unhappy. His peak flows were consistently above normal and he had none of the symptoms that had been reported as being persistently present when he was at home. With his agreement, a progressive exercise programme, based predominantly on swimming, was introduced by the paediatric physiotherapist. Within a few days, there was a dramatic improvement in his mood and his exercise tolerance quickly increased without the appearance of any symptoms. He said that he had never felt better. It was possible to reduce the bronchodilator therapy he received. After close liaison between the hospital physiotherapist and the local community physiotherapist, GP and practice nurse, he went home with a written self-management plan and contact numbers for advice.

Over the next few months, he remained well. He felt confident to participate in some sports at school and his attendance improved. As he needed no oral steroids, his weight fell and his cushingoid features disappeared.

Comment

This child was undoubtedly suffering from severe asthma which was poorly controlled at the time of his referral. However, the anxiety of both the child and his mother were worsening the situation. As attempts to reduce treatment or increase activity simply raised the level of this anxiety, a period of closely supervised and supported admission was arranged. Such a planned admission for the stabilization of asthma in children is rarely necessary nowadays, but it can be very effective in unusual cases.

The involvement of a skilled physiotherapist was vital to increase progressively the exercise David would do and, more importantly, to reassure him and his mother that this was safe, possible and even enjoyable. Close liaison with the local health care professionals was essential to ensure that a consistent approach was maintained after he went home. An agreed written self-management plan aided this consistency.

Cases 3 and 4: Recurrent cough and wheeze

Managing an infant who presents with recurrent cough and wheeze is a common and difficult problem for all health professionals who deal with children. There are many different reasons why young children wheeze, some serious, others demanding only reassurance. Not all that wheezes is asthma in this age group. Over two-thirds of children who wheeze in the first year of life **do not** develop asthma that continues into later childhood. Treatment that works well in older children and adults may be quite ineffectual in this age group: effective drug delivery is also more difficult. The two case histories that follow illustrate some important aspects of the assessment and management of this difficult problem.

Case 3

A 10-month-old boy with recurrent cough and wheeze was referred by his GP to a paediatrician. He had developed eczema at the age of two months and frequent chest symptoms by four months. At first he was not distressed by these symptoms, but for the previous three months his activities, and particularly his sleep, had become increasingly disturbed. Two older siblings had suffered from the early onset of both eczema and asthma and his mother had been asthmatic all of her life.

On examination, he was thriving. There was mild subcostal recession, hyperinflation of the chest with a prominent sternum, and widespread wheeze. Apart from typical infantile eczema, there were no other abnormalities.

In view of the severity and frequency of his symptoms, he was started on budesonide 200 μg twice daily through a nebuhaler and soft Laerdal facemask. He was prescribed inhaled terbutaline for relief. The asthma nurse specialist showed his parents how to use the inhalers and confirmed that he tolerated them. His mother was concerned because there was no immediate improvement on this treatment. She made repeated visits to the GP and telephone calls to the hospital asthma nurse specialist. After three to four weeks, the child's symptoms settled and his sleep pattern returned to normal.

Comment

Although there are many causes of recurrent wheeze in infants, the strong family history of atopic disease and the coexisting eczema in this child support a diagnosis of asthma. The decision about whether or not to treat symptoms depends largely on the degree of distress the symptoms are causing to the child. If there is no disturbance of the child's activities and sleep, and the child is otherwise well, then reassurance of the parents is often all that is required.

This was not the case in this child and the introduction of a trial of inhaled prophylaxis was appropriate. Sodium cromoglycate is usually ineffectual in this age group and is not recommended. Oral bronchodilators are widely prescribed but rarely beneficial. The response to inhaled steroids is variable: even where they are effective, there may be no improvement for several weeks and a trial of at least six to eight weeks is therefore reasonable. The parents should be warned of this. A spacer with facemask is the inhaler device of choice. It is more convenient for the parents and probably more effective than nebulized treatment in most cases. It is also considerably cheaper.

Case 4

A 17-month-old boy, with acute wheeze and breathlessness and a diagnosis of asthma, was admitted as an emergency at the GP's request. The child had had two similar episodes in the previous year which the GP had treated at home with oral salbutamol and a short course of prednisolone. Between these episodes he had been noted to have a moist cough, but this had not distressed him too much. He had three older brothers who had asthma requiring inhaled steroids.

On admission, he was breathless, with moderate subcostal and intercostal recession. There were high-pitched wheezes and coarse crackles throughout the lung fields. He looked scrawny and his weight was below the third centile for his age. The nurses commented that his stools were greasy and offensive.

Comment

There are several aspects of the history and examination that should immediately call the diagnosis of asthma into doubt in this child. The moist cough, the crackles (crepitations) in the chest, and most importantly, the low weight centile, all suggest that there is another cause for the recurrent chest symptoms. The appearance of the stools is suggestive of malabsorption and steatorrhoea.

As cystic fibrosis can present in this way, a sweat test was performed. This showed the raised sweat electrolyte levels diagnostic of cystic fibrosis. The boy responded well to antibiotics, physiotherapy and pancreatic and dietary supplements. Sweat tests performed on his three brothers were fortunately all normal.

Although cystic fibrosis and some of the other causes of recurrent wheeze and cough in the young child are individually uncommon, they need to be considered in children who have unusual symptoms or signs. Failure to thrive is not a feature of asthma: in children with poor weight gain, other causes should be sought. Referral to a paediatrician for assessment and specialist investigation will often be appropriate.

Case 5: Poor compliance, life-threatening asthma and the challenge of the teenage patient

Steven was 13 years old and a regular attendee at the local A&E department with his unstable asthma. He had been admitted with severe acute asthma on 11 occasions in the previous two years. He had needed intravenous aminophylline and steroids in six of these admissions because of the severity of the attack and the slow response to nebulized bronchodilators and oral prednisolone. During each admission, the importance of taking his prescribed treatment of high-dose inhaled steroids, salmeterol and terbutaline was emphasized. His inhaler technique was regularly checked and found to be excellent. He was given appointments for the children's chest clinic, but he never attended. His GP was informed after each admission but Stephen never attended the surgery or the GP's asthma clinic.

On the night of his final admission, he was found severely breathless, blue and drowsy by his mother. He had used a whole salbutamol MDI in the previous 12 hours but had not taken any other action. Whilst being rushed to hospital by ambulance, he suffered a respiratory arrest. He was rapidly resuscitated and admitted to the paediatric intensive care unit. He responded well to ventilation, steroids and frequent nebulized bronchodilators, and was well enough to be transferred to the normal ward after 36 hours.

In the discussions that followed, Stephen and his parents admitted that he had not taken any medication regularly for the previous two years. In addition, Stephen, like both his parents, was a regular smoker: they had made no attempt to discourage him from this. They had no explanation for why he kept none of his out-patient appointments.

The family were told bluntly by the consultant paediatrician that there was a high risk of Stephen dying or being left with permanent hypoxic brain damage as a result of his recurrent severe acute asthma if he did not accept that he needed to take regular treatment. The potential benefits of such therapy were again stressed to the family.

The Specialist Asthma Nurse was involved in all of these discussions. She made regular home visits after his discharge and spent a great deal of time negotiating what the clinicians regarded as the vital aspects of his treatment. Over the next few weeks there was a dramatic improvement in his symptoms and his lung function. With this improvement, Stephen eventually recognized that the distressing symptoms he had tolerated for so long could be avoided. One year after his near-fatal attack, he had required no admissions to hospital and was much happier.

Comment

Poor compliance or adherence to therapy is common in all age groups but is a particular problem in some teenagers. In this case, the result was very nearly fatal.

It is unlikely that such intensive support and encouragement as was offered by the Specialist Asthma Nurse could have been given by a doctor. Home visits were thought to be an essential ingredient in this approach. Under other circumstances, the involvement of a suitably trained practice nurse could have served this purpose just as well, but such a person was not available in this case.

Case 6: Asthma and bronchiectasis

This boy was diagnosed asthmatic by his GP at the age of $8\frac{1}{2}$ years. The diagnosis was based on a PEF variability of 20% (240–300 l/min), a history suggestive of asthma and a strong family history of atopy and asthma. He had had a tonsillectomy at the age of six for recurrent tonsillitis. He had previously consulted with recurrent upper respiratory tract infections, severe episodes of sinusitis and was seen by an ENT surgeon on a number of occasions. He also suffered from hayfever and recurrent dental abscesses. Skin tests were positive for house dust mite, feathers, cat fur and dogs. The family had two cats at home. Chest X-ray was normal when he was 10 years old.

During the next few years, he had recurrent episodes of acute asthma requiring short courses of oral steroids, one of which necessitated admission to hospital in Spain. During this time he was controlled on high doses of inhaled topical steroids and his PEF fluctuated between 200 and 410. He was admitted three times for pneumonia during his 14th and 15th years; a sweat test was negative for cystic fibrosis.

At this point his mother requested a referral to a specialist respiratory physician and this was arranged. He was seen at the Brompton hospital, where the respiratory paediatrician raised the question of bronchiectasis at the initial consultation and this was subsequently confirmed on CT scan (Figure 7.2a), which was in keeping with a diagnosis of basal bronchiectasis of unknown aetiology. His chest X-ray was compatible with asthma (Figure 7.2b).

He is currently (at age 17) fairly well controlled on fluticasone 500 μg bd, salmeterol 50 μg bd, salbutamol 200 μg bd, intermittent courses of cefixime or azithromycin and, of course, physiotherapy administered by the boy himself.

Comment

The main lesson learnt from this boy's history was that a referral to a specialist respiratory paediatrician should be considered in cases of childhood asthma where there are other complicating factors. This boy had recurrent sinusitis for which he saw a number of ENT surgeons, and three hospital admissions to 'general' paediatric wards. Unfortunately, the full extent of his condition was not diagnosed. It was the boy's mother who requested the referral to the specialist because, unfortunately, his GP (ML) had not appreciated the fact that things were not progressing satisfactorily.

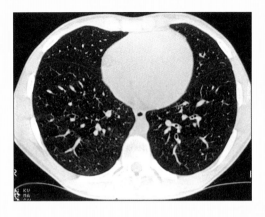 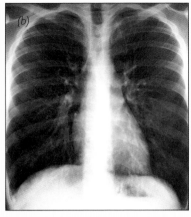

Figure 7.2 *(a) CT scan of bronchiectasis in a child. (b) X-ray showing bronchial wall thickening. (Kindly provided by Dr Andrew Bush, Royal Brompton Hospital, London).*

Case 7: Severe asthma attack in middle age

Annabel had been a heavy smoker when she was diagnosed as a late onset asthmatic at the age of 45 years. The diagnosis was based on wheezing episodes associated with peak flow variability from 200 to 300 l/min (33% variation). She was advised to stop smoking and treated with intermittent salbutamol by inhalation when wheezy. She attended her GP with a severe attack a year after diagnosis for the first time, with a self-diagnosed episode of acute asthma. She had been coughing and waking for a week and presented with severe shortness of breath with a PEF of 130 l/min. Nebulized salbutamol afforded little relief and her peak expiratory flow only increased by 10 l/min. Therefore, admission to hospital was arranged by the GP with the senior medical registrar on call for the local hospital. Unfortunately, the patient was not admitted, because she had a normal chest X-ray and chest examination. The hospital team had not measured her PEF. The patient's peak expiratory flow chart is shown (Figure 7.3) and it is clear that it took at least 10 days on high dose oral steroids to resolve this attack. Her subsequent chart is also shown where her readings stabilized at about 400 l/min.

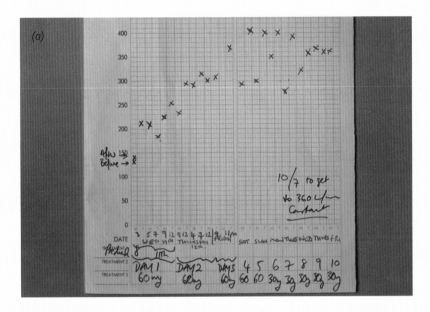

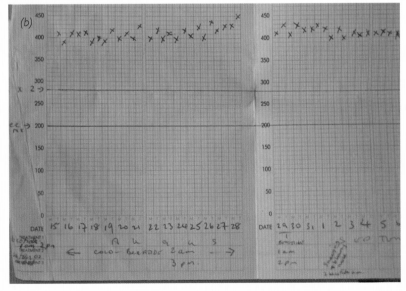

Figure 7.3 *Peak expiratory flow chart showing before (a) and after (b) a course of high-dose oral steroids.*

Since then the patient has been well controlled on fluticasone propionate 1000 µg bd via a volumatic, salmeterol xinafoate 50 µg bd and two short courses of oral steroids for asthma exacerbations.

Comment

One of the most difficult tasks for a doctor or nurse looking after a patient following an asthma attack, is to decide when to reduce and stop the oral steroids. A peak expiratory flow chart is invaluable in these situations. This patient's history also demonstrates that there is a need for adequate training of doctors at all levels in the management of asthma. This particular senior registrar was a gastrointestinal expert — if the patient had had an ulcer, she would have been fine! In fact, in an ideal world, there should be a specialist respiratory team on call, in hospitals, in order to deal with acute asthmatic patients referred by GPs.

Case 8: Asthma in an elderly smoker

A woman aged 66 presented to the nurse practitioner, with two-year history of cough, and a long history of smoking, although she was only smoking one to two cigarettes per month at the time of consultation. She had a past history of eczema. Her PEF was monitored for two weeks with intermittent salbutamol for relief, and this varied from 240 to 280 l/min. She was treated on the intermittent salbutamol for a further month and her PEF varied between 250 and 310 l/min (19% variability). Her chest X-ray was normal, and after discussion with the GP, she was prescribed a trial course of inhaled fluticasone 750 µg bd via a volumatic. Her PEF increased to 360–410 l/min (12% variability) and her cough has improved somewhat. Her flow volume curve performed in the practice has improved since initiating the inhaled steroids. The FVC has increased by 16% and her FEV_1 by 10%.

Comment

In patients with past history of smoking, it sometimes takes a while for the patient to respond to therapy. It is worth persevering as this case shows.

Case 9: Is the diagnosis correct?

A 7-year-old boy was referred to a respiratory paediatrician with 'poorly controlled asthma'. He was receiving high doses of inhaled steroids through an appropriate inhaler but also needed frequent bronchodilators. Repeated short courses of prednisolone had produced little improvement.

A detailed history revealed that he had a persistent cough producing green sputum, and wheeze and breathlessness on exercise. On examination, there were coarse crackles and a few wheezes audible at both bases. A chest X-ray, and subsequently a CT scan of his chest, showed bronchiectasis. Further investigations revealed an immune defect. Continuous antibiotic prophylaxis produced a dramatic improvement in his symptoms and general health, and it was possible to reduce his anti-asthma therapy.

Comment

If children with recurrent chest symptoms that are thought to be due to asthma fail to respond to appropriate treatment, it is important to consider whether there may be another diagnosis. Not all that coughs and wheezes is asthma.

Case 10: Importance of the right inhaler device

A 6-year-old boy was referred to a hospital clinic with a three-year history of frequent cough, wheeze and breathlessness and repeated acute exacerbations of asthma, resulting in repeated hospital admissions and monthly courses of oral steroids. The referral letter stated that he was on regular cromoglycate and beclamethasone pressurized metered dose inhalers (pMDI), slow-release theophylline capsules and regular nebulized salbutamol.

On examination, he was cushingoid, with a height below the third centile. When asked to show how he used his pMDI, it was evident he could not use the device correctly. His parents said that they had never been shown how to use the inhaler, either by the GP or during their many hospital visits.

He was shown how to use a large volume spacer with his pMDI and given beclomethasone 400 μg twice daily, with salbutamol through the same device on an as-required rather than regular basis. His symptoms rapidly came under control; he required hospital admission on only one occasion in the next two years and his growth rate returned to normal.

Comment

If a patient cannot use their inhaler properly, the drug and the dose prescribed becomes largely irrelevant. Teaching and checking inhaler technique is an essential part of continuing care, whether in primary care or the hospital setting.

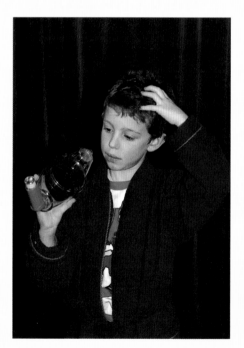
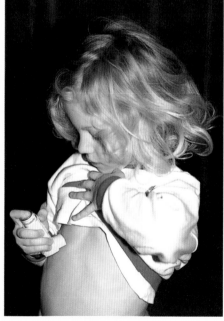

In this case, the child was prescribed a pMDI plus a large volume spacer, which may prove impractical at playtime. A dry powder device (such as an Accuhaler or Turbohaler) may be appropriate for relief medication at this time. However, issuing various devices, in the same child may hinder his ability to use them properly.

Case 11: Avoidable asthma death

During infancy MB had frequent visits to the GP with 'chestiness' and intermittent wheezing. Her mother stated that she was 'never away from the doctor' and 'always getting a cough bottle or antibiotics'. By the age of three years, symptoms had become more frequent and persistent; she was breathless on exercise or when excited and her mother noticed MB wheezing in her sleep.

By the age of four years the family had moved to a new area. After two months, when MB presented to the GP with a chest infection, her history was reviewed and, in the light of intermittent wheezing at night, exercise symptoms and frequent 'chestiness', a diagnosis of asthma was made. MB was started on Intal four times daily. This resulted in a good initial response and she was much improved.

MB was referred to the local paediatric respiratory clinic at the age of six. She was from a deprived social background and her father, who was a heavy smoker and a labourer, had left the family home six months earlier. MB was cared for by her mother who smoked intermittently. During her first year at school she had recurrent exacerbations of asthma relating to infections.

Assessment showed that MB was small for her age, had scattered rhonchi and peak flow measurements showed diurnal variation of 30%, with a 25% fall in the peak flow after five minutes of sustained exercise.

MB was started on moderate doses of inhaled steroids. Her symptoms and respiratory function tests settled, resulting in the dosage of inhaled steroids being reduced. MB was discharged for follow-up at the practice asthma clinic.

MB remained fairly stable until the age of 14 when she was referred back to the adult respiratory clinic with a history of increasing nocturnal and exercise symptoms despite her being on high-dose inhaled steroids. Peak flow measurements again showed a diurnal variation of 25%, with a 40% fall in peak flow on exercise. Her GP had prescribed inhaled steroids through the spacer device. In practice, the patient was taking MDI straight into her mouth. She was able to use the turbohaler effectively and changed onto high-dose budesonide with clinical improvement and lessening in the diurnal variation, but still complaining of morning and exercise symptoms. After starting on a regular long-acting beta-2 agonist (Serevent), MB had reasonable control over the next 18 months but was intermittently symptomatic.

She continued to attend both the general practice and hospital asthma clinics. After discussions between the Consultant and GP the prescriptions for inhaled steroids were checked. MB was clearly not taking the prophylactic medication as prescribed. She was seen by the practice nurse for counselling sessions and some improvement was shown over the next six months.

On leaving school she had poorly paid jobs and could not afford both her prescription charges and to finance her social life. As a result of peer pressure she chose the latter, spending her money on clothes and entertainment.

A few days before the final event, MB developed an upper respiratory tract infection and started using her bronchodilator excessively. She worked in the social club on Friday night as she was going to a disco on Saturday evening. Throughout the day on Saturday her asthma was poorly controlled and she had a poor response to her bronchodilator. MB did not seek medical help as she was keen to go to the disco that evening. After two hours at the disco she collapsed. The GP and ambulance were called but MB had a respiratory arrest in the ambulance. Resuscitation was unsuccessful. MB was aged 17½ at the time of her death.

Comment

Early features suggestive of asthma were missed and only realized when the patient changed practice. A very good initial response to sodium cromoglycate four times a day was seen but once the patient started school this became inconvenient. There were significant social and family problems, plus exposure to infection in the first year at school leading to worsening of symptoms. The patient was referred to the hospital clinic for advice regarding management. During this phase the mother was very supportive and MB was willing to take regular inhaled steroids through a spacer device. In her teenage years conflicts were more common and she was using the MDI straight into her mouth rather than via the spacer. On leaving school the patient experienced major financial, social and domestic problems in addition to having three jobs, two of them unsuitable. MB was not able to cope with the financial decisions in her life. The practice offered as much help and support as possible but the patient failed to attend regularly.

Case 12: Occupational asthma

A 24-year-old man, married with two children (aged two and six months) and a mortgage to pay, who smoked 10 cigarettes per day, was employed as a paint sprayer in the motor trade. There was a past history of bronchitis during the winter months. From his eighth year he was breathless on exercise which restricted gym and sporting activities, although he grew out of this before secondary school. Hayfever developed at age 11 but after age 14 the symptoms improved. As an infant he had suffered eczema and his mother and sister had asthma.

After leaving school aged 16 years, he took a job as an apprentice paint sprayer in the motor trade. He did his training in a well-equipped paint shop using good respiratory protection. However, no pre-employment or regular medical checks were undertaken during his apprenticeship.

At the age of 22 years, following the birth of his eldest child, he was offered a job in a small back street repair firm with much better pay. After six months he began to develop a stuffy nose, particularly in the evening. A year later he began to complain of chest tightness in the evenings and after playing football. He did not bother to contact his GP.

After a further six months he presented to his GP with protracted 'chest infection', stuffy nose, cough, sputum production, chest tightness and breathing difficulties which prevented him from continuing to work. The patient was given two courses of antibiotics to which he was non-responsive and was referred to the local chest clinic for further investigations.

Pointers to the likely diagnosis from the history were the respiratory symptoms as a child, the hayfever and the development of nasal symptoms and chest tightness while working in an occupation known to use respiratory sensitizers such as isocyanates. Widespread rhonchi were noted on examination. The peak flow was only 230 against a predicted 600 l/min. Ventilatory function confirmed obstructive airways disease with 15% reversibility following a bronchodilator. A chest X-ray was non-specific. A RAST test for isocyanates was performed.

The patient was started on 50 mg of prednisolone a day and asked to do daily peak expiratory flow readings. Over the first week there was some improvement but the variation was >25% confirming the diagnosis of asthma. Prednisolone was continued at 25 mg daily and the patient commenced high-dose inhaled steroids.

Two weeks later, the peak flows were stable around 600 l/min. The patient, having been off work since before the referral to the chest clinic, was allowed back to work and was asked to take regular peak expiratory flow readings during the day. By the evening of the first day he was complaining of chest tightness and the peak flow had fallen to 500 l/min. By lunch time on the second day he was suffering from acute breathlessness, had a peak flow of 320 l/min and was certified unfit for work.

Comment

The significance of the history was not realized. Nobody with a history of asthma should be employed in an industry using one of the known occupational asthma sensitizing chemicals, such as isocyanates or collophony. This includes the occupation of paint spraying. The pre-employment medical should have detected the previous history of both rhinitis and asthmatic features. Even if he had slipped through this net he should have been checked at three months and thereafter at six monthly intervals. These guidelines were introduced by the Health & Safety Executive in 1977 and have been law since the mid 1980s.

In a young man with financial commitments such as starting a family, the prospects of higher income led to him changing to a working environment with inappropriate working practices. The progressive development of nasal symptoms, chest tightness and then acute respiratory symptoms is characteristic of many cases of occupational asthma. Often the GP confuses the acute event with an infection. Referral was appropriate and one would expect the specialist physician to note the salient points in the history and initiate an appropriate assessment as indicated.

Keeping the patient away from work and giving oral steroids, followed by inhaled steroids, invariably leads to a fairly rapid improvement. The subsequent relapse following return to work is not uncommon although inhaled steroids may lessen the severity. The extent of the reaction will depend on the level of exposure to the offending agent, in this case isocyanates (even small concentrations are sufficient to cause major problems).

The future needs to be discussed with this patient. If he were working with a larger company he may be found alternative employment where he is not exposed to isocyanates. He should be advised to seek compensation from the DHSS and the question of possible compensation from his employer has to be addressed. There is considerable social impact — he is likely to lose his relatively well-paid job and would not be allowed to return to any employment where he would be exposed to isocyanates. He has a young family and a mortgage and needs advice on these matters. Some patients' symptoms improve dramatically when they change jobs and they require little further support. Others require long-term inhaled steroids with regular support from follow-up.

Case 13: The differential diagnosis between COPD and asthma

A 45-year-old male, having smoked 20 cigarettes per day since the age of 11, worked for many years as a welder in a shipyard. He presented to his GP in late January with a history of increasing breathlessness over a period of three years. He had had recurrent episodes of winter infection usually managed with over-the-counter medications. This year the symptoms were more severe and persistent and were associated with increased breathlessness and wheeze, worse at night and first thing in the morning. He had difficulty in continuing at work. His symptoms had become particularly worse over the past three weeks.

His pulse was 80 and his blood pressure 130/84. Heart sounds were normal. There was diminished air entry with scattered rhonchi in both lung fields. His peak expiratory flow on assessment was 210 l/min. A diagnosis of acute-on-chronic asthma was made and the patient was treated with antibiotics and a course of oral steroids. The patient returned after one week; the acute symptoms of cough and sputum had improved as had his breathlessness. However, he was still significantly limited in his exercise tolerance and was having difficulty walking up the hill from work. His peak expiratory flow reading was noted to be 240 l/min. He was given a further week's course of oral steroid (50 mg prednisolone daily) followed by Becloforte four puffs b.d. through a volumatic.

Six weeks later, his peak expiratory flow was still 230 l/min. His breathlessness was unchanged. He was referred to the local respiratory unit with a diagnosis of late onset asthma where he requested advice regarding further management.

A chest X-ray (Figure 4.3) showed hyperinflated lungs with flattening of the diaphragm and chronic changes suggestive of COPD. Spirometry gave the following results:

	Before bronchodilator	Post bronchodilator	Predicted	FEV_1 as % Predicted
FEV_1 (litre)	1.4	1.5	2.8	50%
FVC (litre)	2.1	2.7	3.5	
FEV_1/FVC ratio	66%	55%	80%	

These results show poorly reversible obstructive airways disease with a significant reduction in the FEV_1/FVC ratio. According to the BTS COPD Guidelines (in press, 1997) the patient has moderately severe COPD, the FEV_1 is between 40 and 60% of that predicted. There is very little improvement in the FEV_1 and in the light of response to oral and high-dose inhaled steroids. He is unlikely to benefit from long-term high-dose inhaled steroids. However, the improved FVC suggests that he should have a reasonable response to regular inhaled bronchodilators. **An absolute improvement of FVC or FEV_1 by 200 ml is considered clinically significant**.

Comment

The clinical presentation does not suggest asthma. There is a progressive worsening in exercise tolerance over several years and there is nothing to suggest the intermittent variations and fluctuations associated with asthma. There is a daily cough and sputum production. The patient is aged 45 and COPD rarely presents before the mid 40s. There is a strong history of smoking — about 34 years. Smoking is the main aetiological factor in COPD. However, the patient is also a welder and there is no doubt that there is synergism between welding and smoking which accelerates the development of COPD. The history of protracted winter infections getting progressively more severe over several years is characteristic of COPD. However, some of the features of the acute presentation such as the worsening breathlessness, cough, wheeze and nocturnal symptoms, can be mistaken for late-onset asthma if the whole picture is not taken into account.

The patient illustrates a poor response, seen in peak flow readings, to oral and high-dose inhaled steroids. While the diagnosis of COPD cannot be made on peak flow measurements alone the readings may be suggestive as in this case. In contrast to asthma, COPD is diagnosed using spirometry. Key measures are the FEV_1 and FVC. The FEV_1 may remain fairly static over six months, but with a remorseless deterioration over time. The majority of patients show only limited improvement of the FEV_1 to inhaled bronchodilators, in which circumstances regular or inhaled or oral steroids will have limited effect. However, the 20% of sufferers who show an improved FEV_1 should be put on regular inhaled steroids. Of more importance is the response shown in the FVC to inhaled bronchodilator, which is characteristic of COPD and suggests a good long-term response to regular inhaled bronchodilators.

The chest X-ray may be helpful in showing some features of COPD such as hyperinflated lungs and flattening of the diaphragm. It is important to make the differentiation between COPD and asthma. COPD requires regular inhaled bronchodilators and inhaled steroids (if steroid responsive) whereas asthma requires regular steroid treatment. The prognosis is also different. **The key to management of COPD is to help the patient to stop smoking**.

A GP or practice nurse should be able to do simple lung function tests within the practice. This would allow them to differentiate between asthma and COPD and to judge the appropriateness of the treatment following reversibility testing.

Case 14: Misdiagnosis

A 25-year-old female hairdresser is a lifelong non-smoker who denies any childhood respiratory problems. She did have eczema as a child and dermatitis four years ago — this was suspected to be work-related. There is no family history of asthma. She attends a six partner practice and over the last three years has been seen by several partners 'whoever was available' for what were described as 'chest infections'. This was diagnosed as chronic bronchitis and she started on antibiotics.

The patient experienced a bit of chest tightness at work when using certain sprays. At the disco each week, she found the smoky atmosphere caused chest tightness and therefore modified her activities. She found it more of an annoyance than a real problem and was not sufficiently distressed to discuss this with her GP.

Later she was playing with some friends when she twisted her back and developed acute severe pain in the lumbar region. Her symptoms had improved by the next day but she still had considerable discomfort. She was seen at the practice by a locum in the evening clinic who prescribed non-steroidal anti-inflammatory drugs which were picked up at 6 pm and two tablets were taken. By 7 pm she was experiencing rapidly worsening breathlessness, symptoms developing over 20 minutes. After a 999 call she was taken to the A&E department of the local hospital where a diagnosis of acute severe asthma was made. The patient was started on oral steroids, nebulized salbutamol and high-flow oxygen. For the next 30 minutes there was no real response — in fact the pulse rate was rising. At this stage nebulized Atrovent and intravenous aminophylline were started together with further nebulization of a bronchodilator.

A chest X-ray showed a tension pneumothorax. This was treated by needle aspiration followed by under-water drainage with subsequent rapid improvement.

Once this acute episode had settled, she was started on regular inhaled steroids. She was referred to the hospital respiratory clinic where advice was given regarding a possible occupational component to the asthma (hairdresser's asthma). She changed her job with some difficulty but following this her symptoms improved. The asthma was controlled with low-dose inhaled steroids and the patient was referred for follow-up to the practice asthma clinic.

Comment

The history was suggestive of asthma; recurrent chest infections with a wheezy basis and a history of eczema and dermatitis. The possibility that the symptoms were occupationally related was not considered, although hairdresser's asthma is a well recognized entity. This is a young woman who has never smoked and therefore the diagnosis of chronic bronchitis is untenable. There is a need to be careful when prescribing non-steroidal anti-inflammatory drugs. There was a clear history of rhinitis, skin allergies and asthma. **These drugs are particularly dangerous if the patient has a history of nasal polyps or aspirin allergy**. Acute severe asthma can develop very quickly from any cause including susceptibility to specific drugs. A poor response to the appropriate management of an acute attack may be due to complications, which in this case was tension pneumothorax. The role of occupational factors should be considered and advice regarding how these may be resolved should be offered, if appropriate.

Referral and discharge letters

Referral

When a hospital referral is deemed necessary, the information contained in the letter from the general practitioner is usually the only information available to the consultant when the patient enters the clinic. It is, therefore, important that this information should be appropriate to the patient's case. A poor referral letter places both the clinician and the patient at an unnecessary disadvantage as might be seen from the following example:

Letter from the general practitioner:

Dear Doctor

Thank you for seeing this 12-year-old boy. He suffers from asthma on and off. On Ventolin but having a lot of wheeze. His peak flow is 250 l/min. Please see and advise.

Yours sincerely

Comment

The general practitioner has not stated clearly what stimulated the referral and the consultant really does not have any idea what is expected. Is the general practitioner in doubt of the diagnosis? Has the boy been admitted to hospital in the past? Is he allergic to any medication or has he any known trigger factors? Are the family able to look after him?

The hospital specialist's assessment of this boy's case:

History
Asthma for 7 years
Missed 10 weeks school in last year
Wakes every night with cough and wheeze
Unable to play sports
On salbutamol syrup (for 5 years) and cromoglycate pMDI (for 4 weeks)

Examination
Marked hyperinflation
Pigeon chest deformity
Peak expiratory flow 50% of predicted value
Unable to use inhaler adequately

Management
Budesonide 400 μg bd via Turbohaler
Bricanyl 500–1000 μg via Turbohaler prn and before sports
PEF chart at home twice daily
Specialist nurse instructs in inhaler technique
Out-patient review after 4 weeks

Comment

■ Inadequate information was provided by the GP about the boy's illness.

■ No attempt was made by the GP to assess impact of illness on the child's activities.

- Inadequate, inaccurate information was provided about current treatment.
- The GP had given inadequate prophylaxis and inappropriate relief therapy as well as an inappropriate inhaler which had never been demonstrated to the child.
- In the specialist's opinion, this consultation in the hospital was not essential for appropriate assessment and management.
- The parents and child reported that they had lost all faith in the GP — they thought that he was not interested and they wanted a hospital follow-up.

To be effective, a referral letter should be comprehensive, with the reason for referral clearly stated. For example, is it to establish the diagnosis and refer back to the general practitioner for care, or does the general practitioner wish the hospital to undertake shared care? Background information is required about:

- patient's asthma
- smoking
- social and occupational history
- concomitant disorders such as eczema, rhinitis or cardiac failure
- drug therapy
- peak expiratory flow measurements made
- treatments tried
- inhaler devices used
- trigger factors if known

A more comprehensive letter on another patient was received by the hospital specialist:

Dear Hospital Doctor

Billy Bond

Thank you for seeing this 4-year-old boy with recurrent coughs and colds. His cough is worse at night and on exertion. Mum has said that he has wheezed on several occasions. He was diagnosed as having asthma aged 18 months and started on Intal and Ventolin via spacers. However, he continued to have recurrent cough and his mother is not keen to change to inhaled steroids as she is not convinced that he has asthma.

PMH
Normal term delivery — Birth weight 8 lb 5 oz
Mild eczema as infant
No family history of note
No smokers or pets at home
Rx Becotide 100 µg bd via Volumatic, and Ventolin 200 µg qds prn via Volumatic

Yours sincerely

Outpatient assessment: History confirmed the above. In the 3 weeks since the referral letter was sent, the parents had given the Becotide as prescribed, with marked reduction in the frequency of the nocturnal cough.

Management
Confirmed GP diagnosis and treatment ideal
Reassurance only — no change in drugs or inhaler required
Checked inhaler technique — excellent as already taught by GP
5 minutes discussion on parents' concerns about inhaled steroids
No hospital follow-up required

Comments

The referral letter provided all the vital information required by the specialist in order to advise the patient and the general practitioner. It was evident that the GP's management was effective and appropriate, but that reassurance about diagnosis and treatment was needed. The parents left the clinic very satisfied with the care from their GP and agreed that hospital follow-up was unnecessary.

Letters regarding hospital admission

When a patient is admitted for acute asthma, there are certain aspects of the nature of the attack and the past medical history that are important. Many general practitioners complain that patients referred to the hospital sector during acute asthma attacks are not admitted. In many cases this could be explained by a lack of information provided by the referring doctor. For example, a patient who has been treated with nebulized bronchodilators before arrival at the hospital may be assessed as normal during the first hour or two post-nebulized medication. Without a detailed letter explaining the particular patient's past asthma history, the nature of the attack and the prehospital treatment administered, the hospital doctor may be forgiven for sending the patient home again.

An example of the details required in an admission letter for a patient with acute asthma is given below.

Letter from the GP:

GP practice details

Date and time

Dear Hospital Doctor

Patient name, address and date of birth

How did the attack start? Any known trigger this time? Duration of attack?

Severity markers:
Poor response to bronchodilators? Waking at night? Can/cannot speak? Conscious level?

Pulse rate? Respiratory rate?

	Actual	Best	Variability (before and after treatment)
Peak flow (%)			

Treatment given:

	Which?	Dose?	Route/device?
Steroid			
Bronchodilator			

Oxygen given by whom?   GP ☐   Ambulance ☐   Not given ☐

Pre-attack medication:

	Dose	Device
Inhaled steroid		
Inhaled bronchodilator		
Other		

Trigger factor:
Smoking history
Social background

Yours sincerely

Discharge letters from hospital staff to the general practitioner

These need to contain information about the treatment and progress while the patient is in hospital. This is often best conveyed in a structured format.

Example of structured discharge letter:

Dear Dr Jones
re Adam Smith (DoB 10.5.91)

Diagnoses
1) Acute exacerbation of asthma; 2) Atopic eczema

Admitted 17.7.95   Discharged 18.7.95

Medication
Becotide 200 µg bd via Volumatic; Ventolin 200–400 µg 4 hourly prn
Inhaler technique checked by asthma nurse
Emulsifying ointment + 1% hydrocortisone

History
Acute asthma attack for 18 hours; triggered by URTI

Asthma well controlled prior to this, with no sleep, exercise or school disturbance. Eczema stable

Examination
Moderate wheeze, hyperinflation and recession. Oxygen saturation 90% on admission

Treatment
Nebulized salbutamol 5 mg 2–4 hourly; Prednisolone 25 mg daily × 3 days

Follow-up
At your request

Yours sincerely

Index

213